CBD Oil
for Health

100 Amazing Benefits and Uses of CBD Oil

Michele Ross, PhD

Adams Media

New York London Toronto Sydney New Delhi

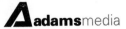

Adams Media
An Imprint of Simon & Schuster, Inc.
57 Littlefield Street
Avon, Massachusetts 02322

First Adams Media trade paperback edition
December 2020

ADAMS MEDIA and colophon are trademarks of Simon & Schuster.

For information about special discounts for bulk purchases, please contact Simon & Schuster Special Sales at 1-866-506-1949 or business@simonandschuster.com.

The Simon & Schuster Speakers Bureau can bring authors to your live event. For more information or to book an event contact the Simon & Schuster Speakers Bureau at 1-866-248-3049 or visit our website at www.simonspeakers.com.

Manufactured in the United States of America

1 2020

Library of Congress Cataloging-in-Publication Data
Names: Ross, Michele, PhD, author.
Title: CBD oil for health / Michele Ross, PhD.
Description: First Adams Media trade paperback edition. | Avon, Massachusetts: Adams Media, 2020. | Series: For health | Includes index.
Identifiers: LCCN 2020014551 | ISBN 9781507213988 (pb) | ISBN 9781507213995 (ebook)
Subjects: LCSH: Cannabis--Therapeutic use--Popular works. | Cannabinoids--Therapeutic use--Popular works.
Classification: LCC RM666.C266 R66 2020 | DDC 615.7/827--dc23
LC record available at https://lccn.loc.gov/2020014551

ISBN 978-1-5072-1398-8
ISBN 978-1-5072-1399-5 (ebook)

CONTENTS

Part 2: Beauty 91

Appendix: Sourcing CBD Oil 120

INTRODUCTION

CBD oil, also known as cannabidiol, or hemp, oil, is a natural plant extract that has been used for thousands of years to promote health and wellness. Filled with potent antioxidants and anti-inflammatories, it is a wonderful tool for both easing symptoms and reducing the likelihood of them occurring. Today, CBD oil is easier than ever to find in local grocery and health stores and online, as more and more people recognize its healing properties. In fact, recent studies show that the benefits of taking CBD oil range from lowering blood pressure and combating nausea, to protecting the brain and boosting your mood. And while CBD oil comes from *Cannabis sativa*, it contains little or no THC (tetrahydrocannabinol), the psychoactive chemical responsible for the "high" produced by smoking or eating marijuana.

CBD Oil for Health offers one hundred easy tricks and step-by-step instructions for putting this amazing little botanical to work for you. With recipes ranging from stomach-soothing shakes and migraine rollerballs, to relaxing massage oils and sleep-promoting tea, you'll find something to fit your health needs, and get a daily dose of rejuvenating self-care—all with the healing power of plants. And CBD oil is just as powerful for the outside of your body as it is for the inside of it: You'll find recipes for beauty treatments that are fun to make and effective. Transform your hair, nails, and skin with DIY anti-aging and healing therapies such as homemade acne masks, relieving sunburn lotion, and moisturizing shampoo for your scalp.

But before diving into the recipes in this book, be sure to take a look at the following section on CBD oil basics. Here, you'll learn more about the history and properties of CBD oil, as well as how to choose the best CBD oil for you. There are also helpful dosing and storage instructions, so you will be able to make the most of each recipe. It's time to rebalance your body and shine from within.

CBD OIL'S MANY HEALTH BENEFITS

CBD oil can seem complex at first. *Cannabinoids, hemp, broad-spectrum, terpenes*: There are a lot of terms floating around when it comes to this little product. You may have never even heard of the endocannabinoid system and why it's so important that CBD oil activates it. Fortunately, this section is here to help. You'll learn the ins and outs of CBD oil—from what it is and its deep-rooted history to the different chemical components of CBD oil and what benefits each offers for your mental and physical health. You'll also take a closer look at the different types of CBD oil, why you might buy one over another, and how to safely use CBD oil. With a proper understanding of what CBD oil is and how it works, you'll be able to confidently purchase your own CBD oil and use it for the health and beauty benefits in this book.

What Is CBD Oil?

CBD oil is an extract made from the hemp plant. Also known as *Cannabis sativa*, hemp is grown across the world for countless industrial and food applications. While CBD oil can be made from any part of the hemp plant besides the seeds, fiber from the stems can also be manufactured into paper, clothing, and rope, and seeds can be processed to create edible products such as hemp seed oil. CBD stands for cannabidiol, which is the most abundant of several cannabinoids found in the oil. You will explore the different chemical elements of CBD oil and their benefits later in this section.

How CBD Oil Works in the Body

Your brain cells communicate to each other with chemical signals called neurotransmitters. The largest neurotransmitter system in the body is called the endocannabinoid system, and is made of chemical signals called endocannabinoids and receptors called cannabinoid receptors. There are more endocannabinoids in your body than there are dopamine, serotonin, GABA, or any other neurotransmitter, and cannabinoid receptors are found in every single part of your body.

The main active ingredient in CBD oil, cannabidiol, actually boosts levels of your main endocannabinoid, anandamide, which binds to cannabinoid receptors and activates pathways that reduce inflammation, pain, and unease. CBD can even activate receptors outside the endocannabinoid system, like serotonin receptors, which regulate key body functions like sleep, appetite, mood, and even sex drive—making CBD oil a versatile tool for restoring balance to the brain and body.

A Brief History of CBD Oil

Cannabis oil rich in CBD (as well as THC) was used medically as early as 1800 B.C., with ancient Egyptian, Indian, and Chinese medical texts referring to it. Moving forward in time, people in the first American colonies and even George Washington himself grew hemp; in the 1800s, England's Queen Victoria used CBD oil to treat menstrual cramps.

In 1906, however, the US Food and Drug Administration (FDA) mistakenly lumped together hemp and cannabis, and labeled them as dangerous and addictive drugs. As a result, medical use of cannabis in the United States sharply declined. The Controlled Substances Act (CSA) of 1970 made cannabinoids (including CBD) illegal, further diminishing its use.

Fortunately, in 1980, Israeli scientist Dr. Raphael Mechoulam found evidence that CBD oil could reduce seizures in children; in 2013, a documentary airing on CNN brought CBD oil into the mainstream media. Recently, the 2018 Farm Bill legalized industrial hemp production and removed CBD from the CSA, making CBD oil fully legal in the United States. Since CBD was legalized, scientific research on it has exploded, with over 2,750 peer-reviewed studies published on its benefits.

The Special Benefits of CBD Oil

CBD oil's unique combination of hundreds of phytochemicals acts on every cell in the body and brain, providing numerous benefits for your mental, emotional, and physical well-being. We'll go over each one of these important chemical properties of CBD oil and describe how it works.

Cannabinoids

Cannabinoids are groups of chemical compounds produced by the *Cannabis sativa* plant; each cannabinoid activates our body's endocannabinoid system differently to produce different health and beauty benefits. Cannabidiol or CBD is one of the more than one hundred cannabinoids that come from the cannabis plant. Despite the name, CBD oil contains many different cannabinoids. The cannabinoids most enriched in CBD oil are the following:

- Cannabidiol (CBD): Making up 40 percent or more of CBD oil, CBD works primarily by increasing levels of the endocannabinoid anandamide as well as activating serotonin receptors.
- Cannabidiolic acid (CBDA): The parent of CBD preserved in some raw CBD oil products, CBDA is effective at boosting mood and reducing nausea.
- Cannabinol (CBN): The THC in full-spectrum CBD slowly breaks down over months and turns into CBN, a powerful sedative and analgesic that makes up less than 0.3 percent of CBD oil.
- Cannabigerol (CBG): Certain hemp strains are rich in CBG, which is nonpsychoactive and has strong antibacterial, anticancer, and anti-inflammatory properties. CBG can make up anywhere from 1 percent to 20 percent of CBD oil.
- Cannabichromene (CBC): This cannabinoid fights cancer and inflammation while boosting brain cell growth—all without the high of THC, and makes up less than 1 percent of CBD oil.
- Tetrahydrocannabinol (THC): The psychoactive cannabinoid that gets you high is not found in broad-spectrum CBD oil or CBD oil made from isolate, which is discussed later in this section. THC makes up less

than 0.3 percent of full-spectrum CBD oil, so it won't have the same psychological effects on you, but will still be effective in relieving pain and reducing inflammation and spasms.

▪ Tetrahydrocannabivarin (THCV): This rare psychoactive cannabinoid is a potent appetite suppressant with the ability to regulate blood sugar and stimulate bone growth, and makes up less than 0.1 percent of CBD oil.

Terpenes

Terpenes are chemicals in CBD oil that give it fragrance and flavor. Each strain of hemp has a different combination of terpenes, creating unique flavors and experiences—as well as additional health benefits. The most common terpenes found in CBD oil are the following:

▪ Beta-Caryophyllene (BCP): A powerful anti-inflammatory, BCP is the only terpene that directly binds to and activates cannabinoid receptors.
▪ Linalool: A major component of lavender, linalool promotes sleep, relieves anxiety, soothes pain, and reduces inflammation.
▪ Limonene: Also found in citrus fruits, limonene fights cancer, soothes upset stomach, boosts mood, and kills bacteria.
▪ Myrcene: Also found in mangos, myrcene is a powerful sleep aid, anti-inflammatory, antidepressant, and pain reliever.
▪ Pinene: A major component of rosemary, pinene opens the airways, increases focus, reduces anxiety, and fights inflammation.
▪ Humulene: Also found in hops, humulene suppresses appetite, fights pain, inhibits the growth of cancer cells, reduces inflammation, and wipes out bacteria.

Flavonoids

Flavonoids make up about 10 percent of the bioactive compounds in the cannabis plant; many flavonoids are present in common fruits and vegetables. The most abundant flavonoids found in CBD oil are the following:

- Quercetin: This anti-inflammatory, antioxidant, and cancer-fighting compound also increases the number of CB1 receptors in the body, boosting the endocannabinoid system.
- Fisetin: This anti-aging superstar combats cancer and increases life span by reducing the number of cells in the body that have damaged DNA.
- Kaempferol: This powerful antioxidant can help fight heart disease, diabetes, and cancer, and can also boost levels of the endocannabinoid anandamide.
- Apigenin: This compound suppresses cancer, reduces inflammation, and can help lower stress levels.

Carrier Oils

CBD and other phytochemicals in hemp extract are absorbed better by the body when fat—such as oil—is present. A variety of carrier oils can be added to hemp extract to make CBD oil; each oil has its own fatty acid profile that influences the absorption of CBD into the body, as well as its own flavor and health benefits. Some brands even combine two or more carrier oils for a unique blend. The most commonly used carrier oils for CBD oil are the following:

- MCT oil: Medium-chain triglyceride (MCT) oil, made from coconuts, is the most commonly used carrier oil for CBD oil. It has many health benefits including reducing inflammation, fighting microbes, and providing energy, and has been made popular by the ketogenic diet. Because MCT oil is comedogenic (it tends to clog your pores), avoid CBD oil made from MCT if you plan to use it on your face and are prone to acne.
- Olive oil: This Mediterranean oil, rich in linoleic acid, provides superior absorption into the skin and gut, is a good source of antioxidants, and has anti-inflammatory properties.
- Hemp seed oil: Full of antioxidants and omega-3 and omega-6 fatty acids, this oil is a nutritional standout that, despite its name, won't add any more CBD to your CBD oil.

- Grapeseed oil: Rich in vitamin E, this oil is often used in CBD oil products for the face because it is noncomedogenic; it won't clog pores.
- Avocado oil: This thick oil, which is rich in vitamin A, vitamin D, and vitamin E, has a nutty taste.
- Sunflower seed oil: This noncomedogenic carrier oil is great to use if you have acne, as it won't clog pores and will actually help to reduce breakouts and improve skin quality.
- Pomegranate seed oil: This oil is usually reserved for CBD oil serums applied to the face and/or scalp to fight inflammation and boost collagen production.
- Emu oil: This animal-based oil provides superior absorption of CBD into the skin and gut, and has potent antioxidant properties.

A Note on Flavoring

The label "unflavored" on a CBD oil product means "without additional flavoring," and has nothing to do with the carrier oil itself. In fact, *unflavored* doesn't mean "no flavor"; it actually tastes like grass. The flavor is most important when using CBD oil under the tongue (if you like mint or orange, etc.) to mask the plant taste, but when it's added to food, the flavoring is negligible.

How to Select, Store, and Prepare CBD Oil

There are many CBD oil products available online, in health stores, and in dispensaries. Some products contain just CBD oil and some have added ingredients. Some are health and beauty products infused with CBD oil. Understanding the different properties and uses of common CBD phytochemicals and carrier oils will help you decide which products fit your own needs. Before you make a purchase, however, there are a few more things to consider.

CBD Oil Variations

CBD is extracted from hemp by using either ethanol, olive oil, or high-pressure carbon dioxide (CO_2) gas. Most CBD oil is made via CO_2 gas extraction, which is efficient but expensive and results in a clear, flavorless extract. Extraction via ethanol or olive oil results in a green extract that tastes like grass. After the phytochemicals are extracted from the raw hemp extract, the CBD oil can be processed further to remove a single chemical or to isolate individual cannabinoids, and carrier oils are added. The following are the three main types of CBD oil:

- Full-spectrum CBD oil: hemp extract that has all of the cannabinoids and terpenes found in the hemp plant (including THC), and contains a carrier oil.
- Broad-spectrum CBD oil: full-spectrum hemp extract that has been processed to completely remove the THC, and also contains a carrier oil.
- Isolate CBD oil: hemp extract containing only the chemical compound CBD, without any other cannabinoids or terpenes, suspended in a carrier oil.

Full-spectrum CBD oil is most effective for wellness applications, followed by broad-spectrum CBD oil, and then CBD oil products made from CBD isolate. If you are hoping to avoid THC completely, it is best to skip full-spectrum CBD oil products and use THC-free broad-spectrum CBD oil products.

Any of the three types of CBD oil can be found in commercial CBD oil tinctures, gummies, teas, patches, softgels, drinks, and lotions, although the least beneficial form, CBD isolate, is used in most brands due to legal restriction on shipping CBD oil products with THC across state lines. To reap the full benefits of all the phytocannabinoids, flavonoids, and terpenes found in the natural hemp plant that are missing from CBD isolate products, it's better to make your own CBD oil recipes at home from full-spectrum or broad-spectrum CBD oil. For more information about how to source CBD oil, see the appendix at the back of this book.

CBD Oil Dosing

There are no one-size-fits-all dosing recommendations for CBD oil, as each product differs in the way it was extracted, the amount of CBD and terpenes it contains, and the carrier oil(s) and other ingredients used. Some CBD oil tinctures have as little as 250 milligrams of CBD, whereas some "extra-strength" formulas have as much as 5,000 milligrams. The standard bottle of CBD oil contains 30 milliliters of product and comes with a dropper that holds 1 milliliter at a time for accurate dosages.

The first step in creating effective CBD oil recipes for health and beauty treatments is to know the concentration of your chosen CBD oil. To determine how much CBD is in 1 dropper of your CBD oil, divide the milligram (mg) amount of CBD by the milliliter (ml) amount in the bottle. For example, if the product label says there are 1,500 milligrams of CBD in a 30-milliliter bottle, each dropper contains 50 milligrams of CBD. Droppers are labeled with quarter markings, making it easy to estimate smaller doses. Once you figure out the amount of CBD in each dropper, look to the product label for more specific dosing recommendations.

This book uses CBD oil doses for recipes based on an average body weight of 150 pounds and normal absorption and metabolism of CBD in the body. A good rule of thumb is adding 1 milligram of CBD oil to your dosage for every 10 pounds of additional body weight. Excessive sleepiness after using CBD oil during the day is a sign you need to lower your dosage, and lacking to see or feel any wellness benefits from CBD oil after taking it for a week is a sign you may need to increase your dosage. CBD oil doses in beauty treatments for the face, skin, or hair do not need to be adjusted for body weight, as they are not absorbed into the bloodstream.

CBD Oil Storage

Always shake your CBD oil before drawing up liquid into the dropper, as the CBD and other active phytochemicals may not be evenly distributed throughout the bottle—especially if it has been sitting for a while. The chemicals in CBD oil can degrade over time and with exposure to light and oxygen, so once the bottle is opened, keep your CBD oil tightly closed in the refrigerator. If your CBD oil is not in a dark bottle, make sure to keep it in the box to block out light.

Safety Precautions

While CBD oil is safer than many prescription drugs, that doesn't mean CBD oil is right for everyone. Ensure a safe, beneficial experience by taking the following precautions before using CBD oil—whether through the recipes in this book or through your own practices:

■ Talk with your doctor before using CBD oil, especially if you have a chronic illness or are taking any prescription medication. CBD oil may not be safe to take with medications that state "do not take with grapefruit" on the label.

■ Always check the label to ensure that your CBD oil does not contain extra flavorings or ingredients that you are sensitive to.

■ Avoid using CBD oil made with MCT oil if you are allergic to coconuts or experience upset stomach or queasiness after taking CBD oil made with MCT oil.

■ Using CBD oil on your skin, hair, and nails is safe while pregnant or breastfeeding, but avoid consuming CBD oil during these periods.

■ Avoid driving or operating machinery if CBD oil makes you sleepy or forgetful.

Over-the-counter medication (OTC) containing CBD oil is not FDA-approved to treat any medical condition. You should not replace proven treatments and medical care with CBD oil.

CBD and You

Adding CBD oil to your daily wellness rituals can be easy and fun. In the following parts, you'll explore one hundred ways to use this natural remedy for your health and beauty needs. Apart from looking and feeling good, you'll also save money by skipping the expensive CBD oil products sold in stores.

PART 1

HEALTH

For so many people, back pain, headaches, upset stomach, sleep issues, low energy, and more are a part of daily life. New treatments and pills crop up every week with promises to fix our symptoms one at a time, while the bottles and costs stack up, and the root causes of these issues are often not addressed. CBD oil contains a combination of potent phytocannabinoids and terpenes, not found in any other natural remedy, that work together to target the different areas of your body and brain, and relieve dozens of symptoms and their causes. In fact, studies have shown that CBD can bring balance to the endocannabinoid system, the largest neurotransmitter system in the brain and body, which regulates the release of all other neurotransmitters. Just 1–2 droppers of CBD oil per day can provide maximal benefits to your health.

This part offers dozens of simple recipes, insights, and bonus tips for using CBD oil to improve sleep, relieve aches and pains, quiet anxious thoughts, and so much more. Take the first steps to restore your health naturally, with CBD oil.

1: COMBATS BACK PAIN

In the US alone, an average of $100 billion is spent each year managing back pain—making it one of the costliest medical expenses you can have. The high prices come from often unnecessary and even dangerous surgeries, injections, addictive opioid painkillers, and alternative therapies like chiropractic adjustments. It would be one thing if these costly treatments helped, but they can actually increase pain and reduce mobility in the long term. In 2017, doctors were issued mandates to stop prescribing opioid painkillers, making a shift to natural therapies like CBD oil a necessity rather than a preference. When combined with a healthy diet and exercise, CBD oil can both reduce back pain and lower the likelihood of it recurring.

Chronic back pain may indicate that your body is out of balance and could even be a sign of endocannabinoid deficiency, which can be remedied by taking 25–50 milligrams of CBD oil under the tongue daily. Phytocannabinoids in CBD oil, including CBD, CBN, and THC, can stop the release of inflammatory prostaglandins that drive back pain. They also activate CB1 cannabinoid receptors that stop the burning, shooting, and stabbing sensations of back pain. CBD oil also reduces overexcitable neurons that trigger muscle spasms. A balm made with CBD oil can also be applied directly to the back for up to 4 hours of pain relief.

TO MAKE AN EXTRA-STRENGTH PAIN BALM, COMBINE:

1 cup organic coconut oil
15 drops frankincense essential oil
15 drops peppermint essential oil
15 drops lavender essential oil
200 milligrams CBD oil

RECOMMENDATIONS FOR USE

Store this balm in an airtight jar for up to twelve weeks. Apply generously to the back, up to 3 times a day. For deeper penetration, apply a heating pad to the area after using balm.

2: BOOSTS NATURAL ENDORPHINS

Many use opioid painkillers, whether it's for a short time to deal with a broken bone, or for months or even years to deal with chronic pain. Because opioids such as oxycodone or fentanyl are highly addictive and carry a real risk of overdose, doctors are reluctant to prescribe them, and encourage patients to use other methods of pain management. One side effect of taking opioids is that your body makes less of your natural opioids, called endorphins, because the medications hyperactivate opioid receptors. When you stop taking opioids, it can take weeks or even months for your body to return to producing normal levels of endorphins, resulting in physical achiness and depression.

One of the ways to recover more comfortably from stopping the use of opioid medication is to boost endorphin production. Meditation, acupuncture, massage, hot baths, and any type of exercise lasting longer than 30 minutes can all raise endorphin levels, helping you feel relaxed and pain-free. It's no wonder why these lifestyle treatments are suggested by professionals for people recovering from opioid abuse. And taking CBD oil can work together with any of these methods to further aid in the natural release of endorphins. The cannabinoids and terpenes in CBD oil not only help relax you, but they also enhance the release of endorphins in the brain.

HOW TO USE

CBD oil works best to boost endorphin levels if you take it internally every day after stopping opioid use. Take 10–25 milligrams of CBD oil under the tongue and held for 30 seconds each morning for up to three months to rebalance your opioid receptors and feel your best.

3: PROMOTES SLEEP

Millions of people are sleep deprived, either not getting enough sleep or getting poor quality sleep. Lifestyle changes such as buying a better mattress aren't an option for everyone, and not everyone can find an extra hour for sleep each day. Prescription medications to treat insomnia come with a laundry list of undesirable side effects such as dizziness, daytime drowsiness, hallucinations, and even memory loss. Prescription and OTC sleeping pills can also become addictive if taken every day, making it hard to quit them even when they stop working.

Most natural methods for insomnia, while inexpensive, are likely to be ineffective. The one exception to this is CBD oil. CBD oil actually works at healing the chemical imbalances or injuries that are disrupting your sleep, rather than acting as a bandage for the issue. CBD oil can reduce symptoms that can cause you to stay awake at night, including pain, anxiety, nausea, and more.

Common mistakes to avoid while using CBD oil for better sleep include not taking a high enough dosage, taking it right before bed (instead of 30 minutes before to allow it to work), and eating a CBD chocolate or other ingestible that contains caffeine. One of the best ways to consume CBD oil is by adding it to hot, caffeine-free tea with milk. The fat in the milk will help your cells absorb more of the CBD oil and the heat will help you absorb it faster.

TO MAKE A BEDTIME CBD OIL TEA, GATHER:

1 bag caffeine-free chamomile or herbal tea
1 mug hot water
25 milligrams CBD oil
½ teaspoon milk (coconut or cow's milk)

Steep tea in hot water for 5 minutes. Remove the tea bag, and add CBD oil and milk. Drink 30 minutes prior to bedtime.

4: FIGHTS IBS

More than 10 percent of the world population has irritable bowel syndrome (IBS), a condition affecting the gastrointestinal (GI) tract that has no known cause but occurs twice as often in women as in men. IBS is not to be confused with inflammatory bowel diseases (IBD)—Crohn's disease and ulcerative colitis—which have genetic components. IBS causes abdominal pain, cramping and bloating, as well as flatulence, diarrhea, and constipation. With no cure for IBS, patients are left trying to manage the syndrome with a healthy diet and stress management. But that doesn't always cut it, and spending all day in the bathroom during an IBS flare-up is no way to live.

Endocannabinoid deficiency is the root cause of IBS, according to neurologist Dr. Ethan Russo. IBS is one of several diseases highly responsive to CBD oil, which restores balance to the endocannabinoid system. CBD oil soothes the GI tract by activating cannabinoid receptors, reducing inflammation and intestinal damage. CBD oil also can ease stress, reducing the chances of an IBS flare-up.

CBD oil can be taken twice daily to help ease IBS symptoms. Each of the ingredients in the following smoothie recipe helps fight IBS:

- Coconut milk: Improves absorption of nutrients into the bloodstream.
- Banana: Restores potassium deficiency caused by diarrhea.
- Spinach: Supplies fiber to keep bowel movements regular.
- Cocoa powder: Acts as a prebiotic, which promotes healthy gut bacteria.
- Peppermint essential oil: Reduces gas and bloating.
- CBD oil: Relieves stomach pain.

TO MAKE A SOOTHING CBD OIL SHAKE, GATHER:

½ cup coconut milk

½ large ripe banana

1 cup fresh spinach leaves

2 tablespoons cocoa powder

3 drops food-grade peppermint essential oil

20 milligrams CBD oil

Blend until smooth and serve immediately or store in refrigerator for up to two days.

5: SUPPORTS BRAIN CELL GROWTH

Children aren't the only ones with growing brains. During adulthood, growing new brain cells, a process called neurogenesis, occurs in specific brain regions, including the hippocampus, an area important for learning, memory, and mood. Adult neurogenesis is involved in many processes, including brain injury repair, cellular plasticity, and maintaining mental health. Many things known to be toxic to your health can reduce adult neurogenesis, including chronic stress, inflammation, alcohol, and hard drugs such as cocaine.

Rich in phytocannabinoids that directly activate cannabinoid receptors in the hippocampus, CBD oil has been shown to promote neurogenesis in adults. CBD oil also contains numerous antioxidants and anti-inflammatories that increase levels of neurotrophic factors that promote brain cell birth and survival. In times of chronic stress, CBD oil can help you relax, which reduces exposure to harmful stress hormones that kill newborn neurons. The following blueberry green tea drink contains powerful ingredients to boost your brain's potential to grow new cells.

TO MAKE A BRAIN-BOOSTING ELIXIR, GATHER:

1 bag organic caffeine-free green tea
1 cup hot water
¼ cup fresh blueberries
½ teaspoon lemon juice
½ teaspoon granulated sugar
15 milligrams CBD oil
1 cup ice cubes

Steep tea bag in hot water for 3 minutes. Remove the tea bag and pour liquid into a blender. Add blueberries, lemon juice, sugar, and CBD oil, cover, and blend until smooth. Pour liquid over ice and serve immediately.

6: RELIEVES HEADACHES

Headaches are a regular part of life for many. While some people are fortunate to have them once in a blue moon, others suffer from headaches weekly or even daily, and they can vary in severity, from minor pain to pain so debilitating that a trip to the emergency room is necessary. There are different triggers for headaches, including hormone imbalances, foods, medications, and stress. Unfortunately, the multitude of OTC and prescription medications don't work for many patients, and the side effects of the medications like severe nausea are worse than the actual headache.

CBD oil is a natural alternative to prescription medications. It reduces pain and inflammation by balancing the endocannabinoid system and relieves stress by directly activating serotonin receptors. CBD oil also opens blood vessels, another way it relieves migraine pain. If you suffer from chronic headaches, it's important to take CBD oil tincture consistently every 6 hours daily or else changes in blood vessel diameter could trigger a headache. Choose a full-spectrum CBD oil that contains THC to get the full benefits, as published studies have shown cannabis containing THC is very effective in reducing migraine headaches. CBD oil is also helpful when applied topically, as it can relieve pain and relax tension in the back, neck, and face muscles that can cause or exacerbate headaches.

TO MAKE A MIGRAINE ROLLERBALL, COMBINE:

5 drops peppermint essential oil
4 drops eucalyptus essential oil
4 drops lavender essential oil
250 milligrams CBD oil

RECOMMENDATIONS FOR USE

Add to a 10-milliliter dark brown glass roller bottle. Cap. Do not use a clear glass rollerball as light reduces effectiveness of CBD oil. Shake before use. Apply to wrists, temples, and back of neck when you feel a headache coming on, and apply every 4 hours until pain subsides. Deeply inhale CBD oil applied to the wrist for extra sinus headache relief. Store at room temperature.

7: TARGETS TUMOR GROWTH

There are few natural remedies that are truly effective at fighting cancer, especially for cancer patients also undergoing chemotherapy. However, studies have shown that CBD oil appears to slow tumor growth, extending the life of patients with certain types of cancers. CBD turns on 680 genes that are anticancer and turns off 524 genes that are pro-cancer, including Id-1, making it one of the most powerful plant compounds known to fight against cancer.

Many cancer cells, like healthy cells, have cannabinoid receptors, and CBD oil can selectively activate or block these receptors. CBD oil can cause cancer cells to die or at least slow their growth. CBD specifically blocks a novel cannabinoid receptor called GPR55; blocking this receptor is associated with slowing tumor growth in colon cancer, breast cancer, brain cancer, and pancreatic cancer. Cannabinoids in CBD oil may also be able to slow cancer cell growth without harming surrounding cells, something chemotherapy and radiation therapy are unable to achieve.

CBD oil holds promise when taken orally and when applied topically. Unlike synthetic drugs, phytochemicals in CBD oil easily cross the blood-brain barrier, where they can fight the formation of tumors in the brain. In fact, a combination of CBD and THC in large doses has been successful in clinical trials to fight a specific and very aggressive form of brain tumor. There is anecdotal evidence collected by doctors across the US that CBD oil applied directly to skin cancers slows their progression and sometimes even shrinks the tumors.

TAKE CARE

Talk to your oncologist about whether taking CBD oil is appropriate for your specific type of cancer and treatment regimen, as it may enhance the growth of some rare cancers.

8: BOOSTS ORGASMS

Using a CBD oil lube can help women have longer, stronger, and more frequent orgasms, according to multiple clinical studies. How? Cannabinoids in CBD oil are quickly absorbed through the mucous membrane in the vagina, activating cannabinoid receptors to increase blood flow, enhance lubrication, and increase sensitivity. Some people even feel the sensation of warmth or of being touched shortly after applying CBD oil to the clitoris. As a bonus, CBD oil contains omega-3 and omega-6 fatty acids that moisturize the labia, as well as compounds that fight bacterial and fungal infections, and soothe irritation.

CBD oil lubricant can be used daily without any negative side effects, as the natural ingredients don't alter the pH or health of the vagina. Store-bought CBD oil lube can be almost $100 a bottle, but you can easily make it yourself for mere dollars with the following recipe.

TO MAKE A CBD AROUSAL OIL, COMBINE:

1 cup softened organic coconut oil
4 drops peppermint essential oil
6 drops organic vanilla extract
6 drops ginger extract
100 milligrams CBD oil

RECOMMENDATIONS FOR USE

Store for up to eight weeks in an airtight jar at room temperature. Warm oil if solid and lightly massage into clitoris and labia 15 minutes before sexual activity. Do not use with latex condoms, as coconut oil damages the latex material.

9: EASES MUSCLE SORENESS

Walking too far, exercising too much at the gym, sitting in front of your computer for the whole day, or having a chronic illness like fibromyalgia can leave you with sore, aching muscles. While one choice might be to apply a commercial menthol balm all over your body, exposing yourself to nasty, pungent chemicals isn't the most pleasant—or cheapest—option. Natural plant-based pain relievers like CBD oil can be effective and affordable.

CBD oil contains several terpenes, including beta-caryophyllene, linalool, myrcene, pinene, and humulene, that relax muscles, relieve pain, and reduce inflammation. CBD, THC, CBN, and other minor cannabinoids in CBD oil can also minimize muscle soreness. One of the best ways to stop all-over muscle soreness is to add CBD oil to a hot bath. The following recipe contains magnesium, essential oils, and cannabinoids that can be absorbed through the skin and can reach deep into the muscles. And as a bonus, you will inhale through the steam from the bath the CBD and essential oils, activating pain relief pathways in your brain. This recipe can do the following:

- Ease muscle cramping.
- Relieve muscle pain.
- Reduce inflammation.
- Increase flexibility.
- Relax the mind.

TO MAKE CBD OIL EPSOM SALTS, COMBINE:

8 cups Epsom salts

15 drops peppermint essential oil

10 drops frankincense essential oil

10 drops lavender essential oil

100 milligrams CBD oil

RECOMMENDATIONS FOR USE

Store in an airtight container at room temperature for up to six months. Dissolve 1–2 cups of Epsom salts in a warm bath, and relax for 20 minutes or more to allow full absorption of cannabinoids.

10: MAKES PAIN RELIEVERS MORE EFFECTIVE

Life can come with a number of pains. From toothaches to burns to back pain to chronic medical conditions like arthritis, it seems like there's not a day when we don't experience some kind of throbbing, burning, or sore pain in some area of our body. Over 20 percent of Americans have chronic pain and depend on taking daily doses of over-the-counter nonsteroidal anti-inflammatory drugs (NSAIDs) like naproxen or ibuprofen, or prescription opioids and antidepressants. Due to overdoses caused by addictive opioid painkillers, doctors are reluctant to prescribe them for anything but acute injuries, leaving patients dealing with chronic pain without many options. For patients experiencing severe chronic pain, NSAIDs just aren't enough, even when combined with other treatment modalities like massage.

Taking just 25–50 milligrams of CBD oil orally each day can bolster the effectiveness of painkillers, without increasing the likelihood of addiction, overdose, or death. CBD oil increases dopamine levels, lessening the desire to use drugs and alcohol and reducing the likelihood patients will overdose on or die from prescribed opioids. Phytocannabinoids in CBD oil including THC and CBD decrease inflammation and pain while boosting mood, which can also help patients reduce their dosage of opioids. In fact, a 2020 study by the University of Louisville found 53 percent of chronic pain patients reduced or completely stopped taking opioid painkillers after using CBD oil for eight weeks, and found their quality of life was improved.

11: EASES ANXIETY

Sweaty palms, racing heart, feeling like you are going to throw up: These are the signs of anxiety almost everyone has experienced at one time in their life. Anxiety can crop up before speaking at an event, during a party where you don't know anyone, or while waiting for the doctor to give you a diagnosis. While it's normal to feel anxiety sometimes, over forty million Americans are anxious most of the time, and qualify as having generalized anxiety disorder. Therapy for anxiety can be expensive and take years to be effective, while prescription medications including benzodiazepines and antidepressants are addictive, difficult to withdraw from once you are on them for years, and have unwanted side effects like decreased interest in sex or excessive sleepiness. Many people also fall back into bad habits such as drinking too much alcohol or smoking cigarettes to manage anxiety. But there is a much healthier way to deal with anxiety—taking CBD oil.

CBD oil is superior to THC-rich cannabis products because, while CBD oil relieves anxiety, THC can trigger it. CBD oil has multiple terpenes and phytocannabinoids that work together to calm the nerves. CBD can directly activate serotonin receptors, which has been proven to relieve anxiety as well as promote restorative sleep. CBD increases the activity of GABA receptors, which helps quiet hyperactive neurons in the amygdala, an area of the brain that manages fear. Terpenes like linalool, also found in lavender essential oil, further help you reach your zen place. While clinical research suggests CBD oil is effective for patients with anxiety, dosing can vary widely from 15–100 milligrams per day, depending on what is causing your anxiety and how severe the anxiety is. Start with 15 milligrams of CBD oil under the tongue once per day and increase as needed.

12: FIGHTS HEPATITIS VIRUS

One of the top ten leading causes of death worldwide is viral hepatitis, which results in severe inflammation of the liver. Viral hepatitis comes in three varieties—hepatitis A, B, and C—and can be either an acute infection (lasting less than six months) or a chronic infection. Most people receive a vaccine against hepatitis A. Over two billion people have or have had hepatitis B in their life. Hepatitis C, which over seventy-one million people have, tends to turn into a chronic infection and may lead to liver failure or even death if untreated. Because many patients with hepatitis show no symptoms, it's difficult to diagnose and treat. Many prescription hepatitis treatments are very expensive, but new research is providing clues about natural compounds that may also be effective against the viruses.

Several phytocannabinoids and terpenes in CBD oil have proven to be effective at killing various microbes including bacteria, fungus, and some types of deadly viruses. A 2017 study published in the journal *Pharmacognosy Research* found that CBD is effective at killing hepatitis C. The more CBD that was taken, the greater the suppression of the virus. Although these experiments occurred only in test tubes, they will likely lead to clinical trials testing to determine the CBD oil dosing necessary to suppress hepatitis C in humans. Talk to your doctor before using CBD oil if you have hepatitis B or hepatitis C, as you will likely need to monitor the health of your liver while using it.

13: MANAGES BLOOD SUGAR

Everything in the body is about balance, and your blood sugar is no different. High blood sugar, or hyperglycemia, impacts millions of people with type 1 or type 2 diabetes. Ten percent of Americans live with diabetes. Symptoms of high blood sugar include increased thirst, fatigue, weight loss, headaches, and blurry vision. If left untreated long term, diabetes can also cause nerve damage, infections, stomach issues, vision problems, and slow-healing wounds. On the other end of the spectrum, low blood sugar, or hypoglycemia, can occur due to treatment for high blood sugar or due to other medical conditions. Symptoms of low blood sugar include confusion, fatigue, hunger, shakiness, anxiety, sweating, and irritability. Even if you don't have diabetes, it's important to maintain a healthy blood sugar balance for your overall well-being.

Multiple cannabinoids in CBD oil, including CBD and THCV, lower blood sugar and improve pancreatic cell health. According to recent research, CBD oil may even help slow pancreas damage in type 1 diabetes if it is used early enough in life. CBD oil can also help reduce appetite and control weight gain, which may reduce the likelihood of obesity, one of the biggest drivers of type 2 diabetes. So, if you're looking to say goodbye to headaches and fatigue, and start living your healthiest life, taking a daily dose of CBD oil could be the ticket to controlling your blood sugar.

TAKE CARE

CBD oil is not a cure for type 1 or type 2 diabetes and does not replace insulin treatment. Type 2 diabetes can be successfully treated through diet, exercise, and medication. CBD oil should be considered a complementary therapy—not a substitute for traditional treatment.

14: COMBATS CROHN'S DISEASE

Crohn's disease and ulcerative colitis are two conditions grouped under inflammatory bowel disease (IBD)—not to be confused with irritable bowel syndrome (IBS). Crohn's disease causes patches of inflamed tissue in the small intestine; patients can experience abdominal pain, loss of appetite, weight loss, fatigue, bloody stools, and diarrhea.

While there's no cure for Crohn's disease, it doesn't mean you have to struggle in silence. Patients searching for an alternative to prescription medications that have dangerous side effects (including developing new conditions like lupus or cancer) are finding hope in CBD oil. CBD oil reduces inflammation and pain in the gut through the following actions:

- Blocking GPR55 receptors in the intestine.
- Increasing levels of the endocannabinoid anandamide that bind to cannabinoid receptors.
- Activating peroxisome proliferator-activated receptors (PPARs) to calm hyperactive immune cells.

Cannabinoid receptors are less functional in Crohn's patients, and require more cannabinoids to activate them. THC oil may also be necessary; studies have reported patients with IBD have improved quality of life after using full-spectrum CBD oil containing THC, whereas THC-free CBD oil appears to have little effect. Talk with a healthcare professional experienced in cannabis care for Crohn's disease before using CBD oil for this disease.

RECOMMENDATIONS FOR USE

Dosing is higher for patients with Crohn's disease than most other health issues. Start with a 30-milligram dose of CBD oil 2–3 times per day under the tongue and allow one week before increasing the dose by 10 milligrams to let the body adjust to it, with a max of 60 milligrams of CBD oil per dose. CBD oil is safe for children with Crohn's disease, and several research studies have found it to be safe and effective in teenagers.

15: SOOTHES ACHING FEET

Whether it's from standing all day at your job, dancing the night away, or having an intense workout session, there's nothing fun about returning home with aching sore feet and calves. Many people also have medical conditions like diabetes or fibromyalgia that make foot pain an everyday occurrence with or without physical exertion. Unfortunately, treating foot pain each day with over-the-counter or prescription painkillers can lead to unwanted side effects like stomach upset, liver damage, or addiction.

CBD oil provides a natural way to treat foot pain in two unique ways: It can be taken daily as a tincture to reduce inflammation and pain throughout the body; and it can be applied directly to the feet for quick and effective relief. CBD oil contains numerous terpenes and cannabinoids that relax tense muscles in the foot to help prevent cramping that can make walking unbearable. The carrier oils in CBD oil contain fatty acids that moisturize the foot, healing calluses or blisters caused by too much walking. When combined with other essential oils, CBD oil topicals can replace certain painkillers.

TO MAKE A PAIN-RELIEVING CBD OIL FOOT CREAM, COMBINE:

$^2/_3$ cup softened organic coconut oil
$^1/_3$ cup aloe vera gel
8 drops peppermint essential oil
8 drops eucalyptus essential oil
6 drops frankincense essential oil
100 milligrams CBD oil

RECOMMENDATIONS FOR USE

Store in an airtight jar at room temperature for up to two months. Apply generously to the top and bottom of both feet whenever sore.

16: ENHANCES ANTIBIOTIC ACTIVITY

Bacteria are ever present in our environment—floating around in the air and lining our bathrooms, kitchens, and even our cell phones. We're in a constant struggle to keep bacteria at bay to avoid getting sick. More and more Americans have been educated on the need to avoid frequent doses of antibiotics whenever possible to forestall both antibacterial resistance as well as the side effects of taking antibiotics like diarrhea.

CBD oil is not only effective at fighting bacteria by itself; it has the ability to enhance the activity of prescription antibiotics by making bacteria more sensitive to the effectiveness of antibiotics. Antibacterial phytochemicals in CBD oil include the cannabinoids CBD, CBC, and CBG, as well as the terpenes limonene and beta-caryophyllene. MCT oil, the most commonly used carrier oil for CBD, also has antimicrobial properties. According to research, CBD kills bacteria within 3 hours of contact. CBD oil can be taken as a tincture, drink, gummy, or other ingestible to fight bacteria and inflammation throughout the body. For targeted antibiotic power, apply CBD oil directly to a cut or infection to kill bacteria and speed healing.

TAKE CARE

CBD oil is not a substitute for antibiotics for serious infections but may be appropriate as additional support. Talk with your doctor before taking CBD oil for this purpose.

17: NURTURES SOBRIETY

Our brains are wired for pleasure, and with the stresses of daily life, many people use negative behaviors to cope such as abusing alcohol, smoking cigarettes, using recreational and prescription drugs, having promiscuous sex, or gambling. Over 30 percent of Americans struggle with drug and alcohol abuse, with many seeking treatment but failing to maintain sobriety.

While CBD oil is often confused with THC-rich cannabis, they are not the same. CBD oil does not cause a high like THC, and in fact, can even help people who are feeling high or manic relax. THC-rich cannabis can be addictive for 9 percent of people, while CBD oil is not addictive and actually may help people who use cannabis and other drugs (and alcohol) reduce their consumption.

CBD oil balances brain chemistry to relieve anxiety and pain that often triggers relapse. CBD oil can help reduce drug and alcohol use, alleviate symptoms of withdrawal, minimize cravings, and keep you abstinent. It also can repair damage to the brain, liver, and even the skin caused by overconsumption of alcohol or drugs. This is due to the antioxidants and anti-inflammatories it contains that fight free radical damage throughout the body.

18: PROTECTS AGAINST BRAIN DAMAGE

Bumps and bruises are part of life, and thankfully, our brain can bounce back easily from most minor concussions. For severe blows to the head, whether it's due to car accidents, sports injuries, or military combat, however, the brain is not so resilient. A traumatic brain injury (TBI) can lead to permanent brain damage or even death. Each year, 2.8 million Americans experience a TBI, and up to 30 percent can require a caregiver to assist them with routine tasks two years after the accident. Anything that can reduce the initial insult to the brain and speed up recovery is needed, but there are few drugs or remedies that can be taken without the risk of negative side effects.

Taking CBD oil each day can be a powerful aid for maintaining a strong, resilient brain. CBD oil contains numerous compounds that act as antioxidants and anti-inflammatories. These compounds reduce free radical damage to brain tissue as well as swelling and pain in the head should an unexpected concussion occur. CBD oil boosts levels of the endocannabinoid anandamide, which protects the integrity of the blood-brain barrier and keeps toxins in the body from entering the brain. CBD, CBC, and CBG are all phytocannabinoids in CBD oil that promote neurogenesis, boosting the growth of new brain cells to repair the injury site. Other cannabinoids in CBD oil promote circulation, whisking away dead cells and toxins through the blood, and bringing in critical nutrients to repair the brain.

HOW TO USE

A dose of 10 milligrams per day under the tongue may protect your brain against damage from injury. Talk to your doctor to ensure CBD oil is safe for you to take if you've experienced a serious brain injury.

19: IMPROVES FOCUS

The average American is easily distracted. And between social media updates, emails, texts, and family responsibilities, it's no wonder most of us struggle with an inability to focus completely on one task. We drink multiple cups of coffee or even energy drinks to stay awake and manage our train of thought throughout the day, but not without harm to our bodies. Caffeinated drinks can burn your stomach lining, erode the enamel on your teeth, cause your heart to race, increase your anxiety, prevent you from falling asleep at night, and cause adrenal fatigue over the long term. Over time, you can also build up a tolerance to caffeine, and may reach for stronger solutions such as prescription stimulants.

Instead, turn to nature and get focused without the jitters by using CBD oil. CBD oil can reduce anxiety, inflammation, and pain, remove distractions and brain fog, and cause your neurons to fire faster. CBD oil also soothes the stomach lining, helping it tolerate more acidic foods and beverages. Some kinds of CBD oil are formulated to induce sleep; they are rich in terpenes like linalool and myrcene, or have added ingredients like 5-HTP or melatonin to relax you. Look for CBD oil formulations that include words like "focus" or "awake" on the label. Make sure to use unflavored CBD oil in the following recipe for the best results.

TO MAKE A CBD OIL FROZEN MOCHA, GATHER:

1½ cups black coffee, cold or at room temperature

½ cup coconut powder

1 envelope hot chocolate powder

15 milligrams unflavored CBD oil

1 cup ice cubes

Add ingredients except ice to a blender and lightly stir with a spoon. Add ice, cover, and blend until smooth. Enjoy immediately.

20: POWERS RUNNER'S HIGH

Athletes often chase that state of bliss, or runner's high, that you get after running a mile or more. For years, this euphoria was believed to stem from an increase in levels of the pleasure neurotransmitter dopamine, while the natural pain-killing effect that comes along with it was attributed to endorphins, your body's natural opioids. Now, a new brain chemical has been found to influence runner's high: endocannabinoid anandamide. Known as the bliss molecule, anandamide binds to your CB1 receptors to reduce anxiety, boost mood, and relieve pain.

Many athletes are known to use cannabis or CBD oil before working out to increase the length and intensity of their workouts. When those CB1 receptors are activated by phytocannabinoids, the intensity of the runner's high is increased. It also relaxes your blood vessels, helping you sustain cardio activity for long periods of time like a marathon. If you need motivation to get to the gym, CBD oil might be the switch that turns working out from a chore into an enjoyable activity. The following smoothie recipe includes maca root, cinnamon, and CBD oil, which all activate your endocannabinoid system to boost runner's high.

TO MAKE A PRE-WORKOUT CBD OIL SMOOTHIE, GATHER:

1 cup ice cubes

½ large ripe banana

1 cup almond milk

½ teaspoon maca root powder

1 teaspoon ground cinnamon

25 milligrams CBD oil

Blend until smooth and drink immediately.

21: SERVES AS A POWERFUL ANTIOXIDANT

Free radicals are molecules containing oxygen that are unstable due to an uneven number of electrons. Antioxidants are molecules that can donate an extra electron to free radicals to neutralize them. Once an antioxidant neutralizes a free radical, it is oxidized and used up until it is recycled and reactivated. Oxidative stress occurs in the body when there are more free radicals in the body than antioxidants. This can cause cell death, tissue damage, and premature aging. Diseases that are linked to oxidative stress include heart disease, diabetes, Parkinson's disease, and cancer.

It's important to limit sources of free radicals like environmental toxins and unhealthy foods, and increase sources of antioxidants. CBD oil contains numerous vitamins, cannabinoids, terpenes, and flavonoids, all with antioxidant power. CBD oil's carrier oil such as MCT oil or olive oil can also be a rich source of antioxidants, or can aid in their production in the brain. Not all antioxidants are the same in terms of how many free radicals they can oxidize and how fast they recycle. For example, CBD is a more powerful antioxidant than vitamin C or vitamin E for preventing brain damage. The United States government even holds the patent on "Cannabinoids As Antioxidants and Neuroprotectants."

HOW TO USE

Adding CBD oil to salads, smoothies, and other meals can boost their antioxidant power, and keep your heart and brain healthy each day. No need to make anything fancy; just add 5–10 drops of CBD oil to any food and mix it in before consuming.

22: EASES MUSCLE SPASMS

Almost everyone has experienced a muscle spasm, whether it's your eye twitching, your back hurting, or your calf cramping up. Occasional muscle spasms can be caused by dehydration, stress, or overexertion, while chronic muscle spasms can be symptoms of serious medical conditions like multiple sclerosis and fibromyalgia. Eating foods rich in magnesium and potassium, and drinking lots of water can help prevent occasional muscle spasms, but chronic spasms are much more debilitating and harder to treat. Prescription muscle relaxants can work to ease muscle tension, but they can also be addictive, and cannot be prescribed in conjunction with opioid pain relievers.

CBD oil stops spasms by activating GABA receptors that inhibit muscle twitching, as well as activating endocannabinoid receptors that relieve the inflammation that causes neurons to be hyperactive. To calm muscle spasms, apply CBD oil that is in a lotion, balm, or cream that is made for pain and contains menthol or peppermint essential oil, otherwise it won't be strong enough for acute pain caused by such spasms. If they know they are prone to muscle cramping, many people use CBD creams twice a day to prevent cramps rather than deal with the pain and muscle injury of having one. To boost the anti-inflammatory and antispasmodic benefits of CBD oil from within, you can also consume 15–25 milligrams of a CBD oil tincture daily.

23: FIGHTS NAUSEA

Acute or chronic illness, pregnancy, chemotherapy, and even stress can bring on queasiness or nausea. Sometimes it can be hard to identify the true cause, which makes it even more difficult to treat. Many people consider nausea to be more unpleasant than vomiting because it tends to last longer.

CBD oil contains several cannabinoids including CBD, CBDA, THC, and THCA that can reduce nausea. Millions of cannabinoid receptors are found in the gut, which is also known as your enteric nervous system or your second brain. When you consume CBD oil, the phytocannabinoids in it activate those receptors, reducing inflammation and pain, and soothing both your gut and your brain. It's best to make your own CBD oil gummies, as most of the ones for sale online or in stores contain chemicals like artificial coloring that can make you sick.

Whisk lemon juice, honey, and ginger together in a medium saucepan over medium heat. Spread gelatin powder on top and whisk continually until mixture simmers. After several minutes, the mixture will thicken, and the gelatin will dissolve. Remove from heat and immediately add CBD oil. Whisk, then pour mixture into an ungreased 8" x 8" square pan. Let pan cool in the refrigerator for 25 minutes or until fully set. After cooling, cut into small squares and store in a sealed container for up to eight months at room temperature.

RECOMMENDATIONS FOR USE

To determine the dosage of CBD oil in your gummies, divide 1,500 milligrams by the total amount of gummy squares you made. Eating 20–30 milligrams of CBD gummies is a proper dosage for nausea.

TO MAKE CBD OIL GINGER GUMMIES, GATHER:

²/₃ cup lemon juice

5 tablespoons pure honey

2 teaspoons grated fresh ginger

6 tablespoons unflavored gelatin powder

1,500 milligrams CBD oil

24: PROMOTES WELL-BEING

Your well-being is like a rating for the quality of your life. If you are happy, healthy, and wealthy, you have a high sense of well-being, but even if you aren't all those things, your wellness levels can still be optimal. Someone who has a chronic or even terminal illness can have high levels of well-being if their mindset is healthy.

CBD oil is unique in its ability to raise the sense of well-being in patients with such chronic illnesses as PTSD, fibromyalgia, migraines, and Parkinson's disease. For patients struggling with pain and depression from dealing with their chronic illness daily, feeling more positive about their diagnosis and life can be a huge improvement. Of course, CBD oil won't zap away all of your cares, but the boost in well-being, from feeling down to okay, or okay to good, etc., is a helpful source of comfort. CBD oil can be taken as 15 milligrams under the tongue to boost well-being, and if you are a regular user but feeling down, you can increase your total CBD oil dosage by 45 milligrams on stressful days.

25: AIDS FAT BURNING

Obesity is a growing problem in many places across the world, including the US. Everywhere we turn, fast food options call our name, and with so much to do each day, we are tempted to pick easy, quick meals that are full of sugar and other unhealthy additives. Thankfully, CBD oil's combination of healthy fats, terpenes, and powerful phytocannabinoids all work together to optimize fat burning.

Fat cells are called adipocytes, and come in two types: white and brown. White fat cells hold a single fat droplet; brown fat cells contain many fat droplets, as well as mitochondria (the energy producers of the cell). Because brown fat cells have mitochondria, they can produce heat and become active when we are exposed to the cold. Fat-burning can occur when these existing brown adipocytes are activated, or when white adipocytes turn into brown adipocytes when exposed to cold, a process called browning. The journal *Molecular and Cellular Biochemistry* found that CBD can kickstart both forms of fat burning.

Of the many CBD carrier oils that promote fat-burning, MCT oil (made from coconut oil) is the best option for this purpose. Research suggests taking CBD oil made with MCT oil before you exercise may help you burn more fat than carbs for energy. CBD oil made with MCT oil may also be more effective at promoting weight loss in general than CBD oil made with olive oil or other carrier oils. Drizzle CBD oil onto your vegetables each day to get a fast energy boost that helps you burn fat and feel your best.

26: LENGTHENS ATTENTION SPAN

In today's overstimulating, media-driven culture, the average attention span has fallen to just 8 seconds. It's harder for us to decide what is worth our attention, and things that aren't novel or particularly eye-catching can be boring. For some people, issues with focus and attention are so severe that they qualify for a diagnosis of attention deficit hyperactivity disorder (ADHD) or attention deficit disorder (ADD). Over 5 percent of Americans have this disorder, and unfortunately, the prescription medications for ADHD can be dangerously addictive, with side effects that include weight loss, jitters, irritability, and insomnia.

CBD oil contains hundreds of plant compounds that work together to rebalance brain chemistry. Phytocannabinoids in CBD oil, including CBD and THC, can help boost levels of dopamine and serotonin—the neurotransmitters that encode what rewards we should pay attention to and be motivated to obtain—that improve attention span and alertness. Pinene, a terpene found in CBD oil, can also increase focus. CBD oil can be used as a way to be more present in your daily life. Some people take 10–15 milligrams of CBD oil added to their coffee each morning as a way to increase attention and performance at work.

TAKE CARE

CBD oil may interact with some medications for ADHD. Consult your physician before taking CBD oil.

27: EASES MENOPAUSE SYMPTOMS

Women are living longer than ever after menopause, and over fifty million women in America are postmenopausal. Menopause occurs one year after the last menstrual period and is preceded by a large drop in estrogen production and decrease in fertility. Symptoms of menopause include irregular periods, mood swings, hot flashes during the day, night sweats during sleep, vaginal dryness, decreased sex drive, slowed metabolism, weight gain, and trouble concentrating. Many women receive prescription treatments, including antidepressants and hormone replacement therapy (HRT), to combat the symptoms of menopause, but these drugs can cause a long list of side effects, including blood clots, nausea, headaches, and further loss of sex drive. Women who also have a history of breast cancer or blood clots cannot use HRT.

CBD oil can balance hormones, boost dopamine, serotonin, and oxytocin, and enhance life long after menopause—without uncomfortable or dangerous side effects. This simple recipe for a hormone-balancing CBD tea can do the following:

- Reduce number and severity of hot flashes.
- Decrease frequency of headaches.
- Ease nausea symptoms.
- Promote quality sleep.
- Boost mood.
- Enhance vaginal lubrication.

TO MAKE A HORMONE-BALANCING TEA, GATHER:

1 bag raspberry and black cohosh tea
1½ cups hot water
25 milligrams CBD oil
1 cup soy milk

Steep tea in hot water for 5 minutes. Remove the tea bag, and add CBD oil and milk. Drink daily during menopause.

28: RELIEVES ARTHRITIS PAIN

Millions of people worldwide suffer from arthritis, a debilitating chronic condition that causes pain and inflammation in the joints. And with multiple types of arthritis out there, including rheumatoid arthritis and osteoarthritis, arthritis can strike patients of any age. The severity and widespread nature of arthritis pain mean that many sufferers are dependent on prescription steroids, antidepressants, and opioids to manage their pain. These treatments have the risks of being addictive, and causing serious side effects like respiratory depression or liver damage.

Unlike opioid painkillers, phytocannabinoids in CBD oil target the root of the problem and don't have dangerous side effects. Beta-caryophyllene and myrcene, two terpenes found in full- or broad-spectrum CBD oil, are popular among patients with arthritis because of their ability to reduce pain flare-ups. CBD oil works best to reduce pain and inflammation when applied topically to aching joints as well as taken under the tongue 2–3 times a day. You can even add CBD oil to every meal, sneaking it into sauces and dressings, as a way to feel less pain. The following Asian salad dressing recipe contains the potent anti-inflammatories of garlic, ginger, and CBD oil—all ingredients that have been clinically proven to reduce arthritis pain.

TO MAKE A CBD OIL SALAD DRESSING, COMBINE:

½ cup olive oil

¼ cup rice vinegar

2 tablespoons tamari gluten-free soy sauce

1 clove garlic, peeled and minced

2 tablespoons grated fresh ginger

30 milligrams CBD oil

RECOMMENDATIONS FOR USE

Store in an airtight container in the refrigerator for up to two weeks.

29: REDUCES FREQUENCY OF SEIZURES

Over three million Americans have a seizure disorder, which can be caused by genetic disorders, brain infections, brain injury, and other medical conditions. Because seizures can cause a burst of brain activity, frequent or severe seizures can cause damage to the brain or require hospitalization if they don't stop. While many patients control their seizures through prescription medications, others have to constantly rotate drugs or dosing, and fail to find something that works for the long term.

The potential for full-spectrum CBD oil as a natural remedy to calm hyperactive neurons and reduce seizures was first brought to light in the CNN documentary *WEED*, produced by Dr. Sanjay Gupta in 2013. As the film detailed, there are several mechanisms for how the phytocannabinoids and terpenes in CBD oil may help to reduce frequency of seizures in children and adults with epilepsy, autism, and other disorders. Antioxidants and phytocannabinoids in CBD oil also calm free radical damage and inflammation in the brain, preventing further damage to sensitive neurons. A 2017 study from the University of Washington found that CBD blocks an atypical cannabinoid receptor called GPR55 and is one of the ways CBD oil reduces the frequency and severity of seizures in a common form of epilepsy called Dravet syndrome. The dose of CBD oil required to reduce seizures is at least 100–250 milligrams per day.

TAKE CARE

CBD oil inhibits the breakdown of several drugs prescribed for epilepsy and may cause a serious drug interaction. Do not begin using oral CBD oil at any dose until you have consulted your doctor.

30: BOOSTS WORKOUT RECOVERY

Whether you're just starting to work out or you're pushing the limits of your endurance, exercise can be painful. Small muscle tears from lifting weights or sore muscles from running can tempt you to skip the gym for a day, week, or even longer. While the expression no pain, no gain rings true at the gym, you don't have to recover in pain at home. There are numerous natural remedies to speed up workout recovery, but CBD oil has emerged as the ingredient both amateur and professional athletes prefer. Unlike THC-containing cannabis, CBD oil has been cleared by the World Anti-Doping Agency (WADA) for athletes to use. Some organizations, such as the NBA and NFL, continue to prohibit oral CBD oil use, so it's best to check with your local sports organizations.

CBD oil contains numerous phytocannabinoids, terpenes, and flavonoids that promote muscle recovery and pain relief after a workout. Vigorous exercise increases breathing and causes oxidative stress in the body. Antioxidants in CBD oil fight oxidative stress, which reduces inflammation and helps muscles heal faster. By fighting pain, the phytocannabinoids in CBD oil can help you beat postworkout fatigue.

Getting into deep sleep can also promote faster muscle recovery, and multiple cannabinoids and terpenes in CBD oil like linalool and myrcene promote sleep. Incorporating CBD oil into your daily regimen on both workout and nonworkout days is key to getting the best results from exercising and feeling your best.

HOW TO USE

CBD oil at a dose of 15–25 milligrams should be taken as a tincture or drink after a workout, not before, so that muscle tissue can properly break down during exercise to be rebuilt again. CBD oil can also be used as a topical and applied to any sore muscles every 4 hours. CBD lotions with menthol or peppermint essential oil work the best for postworkout pain.

31: INVITES PLEASANT DREAMS

Nightmares don't just happen to people who've watched a scary movie before going to sleep. Many medical conditions involving the brain (including post-traumatic stress disorder, bipolar disorder, and Parkinson's disease), as well as side effects of different medications can cause terrifying vivid dreams. Nightmares can cause tossing, turning, and even screaming in your sleep, making it impossible for you to get a good night's sleep, and even scary for a partner to sleep near you. Unfortunately, turning to prescription medications to reduce symptoms can leave you feeling groggy in the morning, and they often do little to help.

CBD oil activates the endocannabinoid system to help you forget scary memories and stop nightmares. In fact, several studies have found THC and CBD to be effective for improving sleep and reducing nightmares in patients with PTSD and Parkinson's disease. CBD oil activates serotonin receptors, promoting relaxation and easing insomnia. With CBD oil, you have a natural and inexpensive remedy for nightmares with few side effects.

HOW TO USE

Take 15–25 milligrams of CBD oil under the tongue 30 minutes prior to sleep each night. Look for CBD oil rich in the terpenes linalool or myrcene to further reduce movement and promote deep sleep.

32: SUPPRESSES APPETITE

Eating delicious, readily available high-calorie food leads many Americans to struggle with weight gain. Lowering the number of calories you eat is the quickest path to weight loss, but diets are a tricky business. They can be a test of emotional endurance, as days of hunger make you irritable and obsessed with the food you can't eat. Most diets also end early with the dieter binging on a forbidden food. Some dieters even turn to unhealthy prescriptions and over-the-counter weight loss pills containing stimulants or untested compounds that can harm the heart, liver, and gut.

While few natural remedies are effective at suppressing appetite, regular use of CBD oil has emerged as a weight loss aid. Unlike THC-containing cannabis, CBD oil does not increase appetite. In fact, CBD oil balances the endocannabinoid system, activating dopamine and serotonin receptors, which reduces the need to compulsively eat or crave sugar. It also contains a terpene called humulene, which suppresses appetite; it can help you lose weight or, at the very least, avoid putting on more pounds. Full-spectrum CBD oil also contains small amounts of the phytocannabinoid THCV, which has been proven to be a potent weight loss aid.

When anxious or under chronic stress, some people become emotional eaters, turning to food as a solace during difficult times. CBD oil activates serotonin and CB1 receptors, boosting mood and reducing the need for comfort food. Add 10–15 milligrams of CBD oil to two meals each day to help control your appetite and stay committed to your diet.

33: FIGHTS FATIGUE

While some people are sleepy during the day simply because they have not gotten enough rest, others can have a solid 8 hours of sleep and yet still wake up tired—or get fatigued later in the day without much exertion. Medical conditions like sleep apnea, fibromyalgia, asthma, multiple sclerosis, and chronic fatigue syndrome (CFS) can all cause fatigue, which is usually the one symptom hardest to treat with pharmaceutical drugs. Many patients with chronic illness turn to THC-rich cannabis to deal with pain, but the phytocannabinoid THC actually increases dizziness and sleepiness, making it a poor fit for their lifestyle.

CBD oil can be applied as a topical to any sore or painful muscles to relieve chronic pain and fight fatigue brought on by these aches and pains, but it's also useful when taken as a tincture or drink. Because CBD oil contains little or no THC, it actually can increase alertness and energy when taken orally in the morning. When taken at night, it can relieve anxiety and promote deep sleep, helping reduce morning grogginess. If CBD oil makes you sleepy when you take it during the day, reduce your dosage, or take it only at night. The ingredients in the following drink work to clear your mind and provide an energy boost, making it a perfect morning beverage for those who deal with daily fatigue.

TO MAKE A CBD ENERGY DRINK, GATHER:

½ cup coconut milk

1 cup no pulp orange juice

2 drops food-grade peppermint essential oil

15 milligrams CBD oil

Blend until smooth and serve immediately.

RECOMMENDATIONS FOR USE

Enjoy within 30 minutes of combining.

34: NURTURES HEALTHY KIDNEYS

Filtering excess waste and fluids from your blood is the job of your kidneys—a pair of organs vital to your health. Kidneys can be damaged by high blood pressure, diabetes, injury, or numerous lifestyle choices, and can sometimes even require kidney dialysis or transplant. Chronic kidney disease (CKD) is common yet often untreated, with 14 percent of Americans having the condition.

Chock-full of antioxidants and anti-inflammatories that help protect against cellular damage, CBD oil can be a robust defense against kidney damage. MCT oil found in CBD oil is full of omega-3 fatty acids that reduce inflammation and reduce scar tissue formation in the kidneys. Cannabinoids in CBD oil can activate two types of cannabinoid receptors, CB1 and CB2, that are found in kidney tissue, and can reduce neuropathic pain from kidney damage by 30 percent. CBD oil can also minimize the effect that unhealthy habits (like consuming sugar and smoking) have on your kidney health; it can balance blood sugar and even assist some users in reducing the number of cigarettes they smoke. Taking 10 milligrams of CBD oil twice a day under the tongue may help promote healthy kidneys.

TAKE CARE

If you are at risk for kidney disease, it's important to avoid smoking marijuana, as it can enhance the decline of kidney function. Taking CBD oil may be an appropriate alternative as it can promote kidney health. Consult your doctor before using CBD oil.

35: EASES FIBROMYALGIA MALAISE

Fibromyalgia is a chronic pain disorder with no known cause. To summarize how it feels, imagine having the flu—every single day of your life. Some days are better than others, but the fatigue, muscle spasms, aches and pains, brain fog, headaches, insomnia, nausea, and depression of the worst days drain your health and happiness. Fibromyalgia is hard to treat because of these many symptoms; patients are often given one prescription for each symptom, which puts them at greater risk for drug interactions, as well as for a laundry list of side effects. Most of the medications are ineffective at helping fibromyalgia patients because they attempt to merely mask the symptoms rather than treat the underlying causes.

CBD oil has emerged as a natural aid for fibromyalgia. Because phytocannabinoids in CBD oil rebalance the endocannabinoid system (the largest neurotransmitter system that regulates all other neurotransmitters in the body), CBD oil can improve much of the malaise fibromyalgia patients feel. CBD oil is highly effective at restoring quality sleep and relieving stress, which can reduce flare-ups of fibromyalgia malaise and improve quality of life. CBD oil reduces inflammation, making a daily CBD oil ritual important for more pain-free days without the grogginess of prescription painkillers.

HOW TO USE

Choose full-spectrum CBD oil, as it contains a small amount of THC that is more effective at alleviating pain and addressing other health issues including muscle spasms and nausea. A standard dose for fibromyalgia malaise is 25–50 milligrams of CBD oil twice a day. If CBD oil makes you sleepy, skip the morning dose. Check with your doctor to make sure CBD oil won't interact with your medications before starting a daily regimen. Topical CBD oils can also be applied to the skin to improve muscle soreness, stiffness, and spasms, without any concern for drug interactions.

36: ASSISTS WITH QUITTING SMOKING

If you've struggled to try to quit smoking, you're not alone. Over forty million Americans smoke cigarettes, and 70 percent want to quit. Cigarettes are highly addictive, and smokers that attempt to quit without joining a smoking cessation program fail an estimated 95 percent of the time. Using nicotine replacement patches or chewing nicotine gum can help some smokers quit, but don't work for others. Cigarette smoking has long-term effects on your health, so the sooner you can quit successfully, the better it is for your health. Some of the harms of smoking include increased risk of lung, mouth, throat, esophagus, and pancreatic cancer; diabetes, heart disease, and stroke; and chronic obstructive pulmonary disease (COPD).

Fortunately, CBD oil has emerged as a potential way to support smokers who are trying to quit. A research study published in the journal *Addictive Behaviors* found that smokers who used an inhaler containing CBD reduced the number of cigarettes they smoked by 50 percent. And while no research has directly studied whether taking CBD oil will have the same impact on people trying to quit smoking cigarettes entirely, there are some early signs CBD oil can help. CBD oil can do the following:

- Reduce stress that triggers craving for cigarettes.
- Boost levels of dopamine and serotonin that are lower during nicotine withdrawal.
- Relieve anxiety that is often the root cause of self-medication with cigarettes.

HOW TO USE

Do not use CBD oil lotion or creams, as they will not be absorbed into your bloodstream and will not help you quit smoking. To maximize your success, take 1 dropper of CBD oil tincture 2–3 times per day.

37: REDUCES AMYLOID PLAQUES IN THE BRAIN

More than five million Americans have Alzheimer's disease, the most common form of dementia that affects seniors. Alzheimer's features progressive loss of memory and cognitive function, and most patients require full-time care toward the later stages. A deficiency in acetylcholine, a neurotransmitter that modulates decision-making and memory, is the root cause of Alzheimer's disease. Another facet of the disease is the development of beta-amyloid plaques in the brain, which are essentially large clumps of protein that cause inflammation and prevent communication between neurons.

Clinical research has shown that preventing formation of beta-amyloid plaques seems to slow progression of the disease. Lifestyle changes, including adopting a Mediterranean diet and eating fewer processed foods, appear to keep the brain healthy and reduce the development of beta-amyloid plaques. Additionally, studies suggest CBD oil is a new tool in the fight against Alzheimer's disease. Cannabinoids in full-spectrum CBD oil, including THC, were found to actively reduce beta-amyloid clumps in the brain. In addition, long-term treatment with CBD oil can improve some memory deficits.

HOW TO USE

Taking 15–25 milligrams of CBD oil daily starting in midlife may promote brain health. Taking CBD oil prior to the onset of Alzheimer's symptoms is optimal, as it is always easier to prevent it than to treat it.

38: TACKLES HIGH BLOOD PRESSURE

High blood pressure (or hypertension) is one of the most common medical conditions in the United States. One in three adults has hypertension, yet only half of them have their high blood pressure under control. Many people take medications to lower their blood pressure, but either forget to take it daily or engage in lifestyle choices that contribute to high blood pressure. You are at greater risk for high blood pressure if you do the following:

■ Drink alcohol heavily.
■ Smoke or vape tobacco.
■ Eat a diet high in salt and/or fat.
■ Don't exercise regularly.
■ Are obese.

CBD oil can help you lower your blood pressure naturally in a myriad of ways. CBD oil can relax blood vessels, which promotes blood flow and lowers blood pressure. CBD oil can also help relieve stress and reduce anxiety, which lowers blood pressure. A study published in the journal *JCI Insight* found a single dose of CBD oil can lower blood pressure under stress. Finally, people who use CBD oil tend to smoke fewer cigarettes and drink less alcohol, further lowering the risk for high blood pressure. Combine CBD oil with potassium-rich foods such as bananas to boost its ability to lower blood pressure. The following recipe is a wonderful and delicious way to lower blood pressure naturally.

TO MAKE A CBD OIL SMOOTHIE, GATHER:

1½ large ripe bananas
¾ cup almond milk
15 milligrams CBD oil
½ teaspoon ginger paste
1 tablespoon pure honey
½ cup ice cubes

Blend until smooth and serve immediately or store covered in refrigerator for up to two days.

TAKE CARE

Talk to your doctor about taking CBD oil if you are taking medication to lower your high blood pressure or already live with low blood pressure.

39: IMPROVES EFFICACY OF CHEMOTHERAPY

Chemotherapy is an intense treatment that kills cancer while making the patient sick. Patients undergoing chemotherapy experience nausea and vomiting, reduced appetite, headaches, pain, and exhaustion. They lose weight, have a suppressed immune system, and fall sick easily. For some patients, chemotherapy treatment does not work to kill cancer cells, or the treatment is too much. For aggressive cancers, the chances of surviving one, five, or ten years after chemotherapy can be slim.

High doses of CBD oil may work to kill certain types of cancer cells. In fact, research published in the journal *Oncogene* found that survival from pancreatic cancer tripled when CBD was used in addition to chemotherapy treatment. It is not clear yet whether CBD oil taken at lower wellness doses, such as 10–50 milligrams under the tongue per day, has any beneficial effect on killing cancer cells.

CBD oil can help make chemotherapy more effective or at least tolerable for patients. It reduces pain and inflammation associated with both cancer and chemotherapy treatment. Cannabinoids in CBD oil, including CBD, CBA, THC, and THCA, have been found to reduce nausea and vomiting, and promote appetite, helping patients maintain their body weight. CBD oil can also improve depression and reduce anxiety around chemotherapy treatment and cancer diagnosis, reducing stress hormones and increasing the patient's odds of survival.

TAKE CARE

CBD oil can inhibit certain liver enzymes that break down medication, including some forms of chemotherapy. It may also cause liver damage at very high dosages or in patients with compromised livers. CBD oil is not a substitute for chemotherapy but may be appropriate as a wellness support. Talk with your doctor before using CBD oil.

40: CREATES RELAXING MOCKTAILS

Over 50 percent of Americans reported drinking alcohol at least once a month, with 26 percent reporting binge drinking. Many people are looking to cut down on their drinking, skip the hangover, and connect with themselves and others instead of tuning out. Drinking less alcohol can also have health benefits such as weight loss, reduced inflammation, fewer headaches, and improved skin.

Regular CBD oil users note that they drink less alcohol without even trying, and several studies confirm that CBD can reduce alcohol use as well as reduce cravings for alcohol in those trying to maintain sobriety. Incredibly, CBD may even repair brain and liver damage from past alcohol use. CBD oil can be a great way to relax after a long day of work. It doesn't matter whether it's taken as a gummy, tincture, or drink, or even used in a vape pen; the end result is a blissful calm. Substitute 25 milligrams of CBD oil for one alcoholic drink.

TO MAKE CBD PALOMA MOCKTAILS, GATHER:

2 cups 100 percent red grapefruit juice
½ cup lime juice
2 tablespoons granulated sugar
2½ cans CBD sparkling soda
Ice to fill

Mix the grapefruit juice, lime juice, and sugar in a cocktail shaker. Divide the sparkling soda between six cocktail glasses filled with ice. Pour $^1/_6$ of the shaker mix into each glass.

RECOMMENDATIONS FOR USE

This recipe makes 6 servings. Chill leftover drink mix without ice in an airtight container in the refrigerator for up to two days.

41: REDUCES AGE-RELATED AGITATION

Aging gracefully can be difficult due to the fact that degeneration of the brain can lead to memory loss and confusion. More than 5 percent of people over the age of sixty worldwide have dementia, with Alzheimer's disease being the primary cause. Many elderly patients require full-time care by family members or senior care staff to help them keep calm and content. Yet due to dementia, they can act aggressively toward their caretakers, behavior that tends to worsen over the course of the day in a phenomenon called sundowning. This aggression can be draining for both patients and caretakers. Because most seniors already are on multiple medications, taking additional drugs to sedate them could lead to unwanted side effects or even deadly drug interactions.

CBD oil offers a natural way for elderly patients to relax. In one of the largest CBD oil research studies in humans to date, a Phase 2 clinical trial finishing in 2020 is testing how full-spectrum CBD oil alleviates agitation related to dementia in sixty patients. This research suggests the number of CB1 receptors in the brain decreases with age and may underlie the age-related cognitive dysfunction that occurs. CBD oil can improve the health of the aging brain by increasing anandamide in the brain, activating CB1 receptors, and protecting neurons from cell damage and death. CBD oil activates serotonin receptors, causing relaxation as well as promoting sleep without the dizziness or high of THC products. Taking 15–30 milligrams of CBD oil 2–3 times per day may be key to comforting aging loved ones.

42: LESSENS MORNING SICKNESS

Almost eight in ten women experience morning sickness during pregnancy. This nausea and vomiting can range from minor, to completely debilitating, where the woman can't work or rapidly loses weight from not eating. In any case, morning sickness is an awful experience that pregnant women look to treat as quickly and as effectively as possible. Unfortunately, some medications that reduce nausea are not safe to take during pregnancy, leaving women depending on expensive, ineffective, or even potentially dangerous medications.

While pregnant women use natural remedies like ginger to aid with morning sickness, they usually aren't potent enough to completely control it. CBD oil without THC is a safe and natural aid for expectant mothers. Terpenes and cannabinoids including CBD and CBDA are effective at reducing nausea and vomiting, and restoring appetite. While THC is more effective than CBD at managing nausea, do not use full-spectrum CBD oil that contains THC while pregnant; THC is able to pass through the placenta and affect the growth of your child.

HOW TO USE

Choose broad-spectrum, THC-free CBD oil, using the lowest possible dose and frequency to manage your nausea and vomiting. Find a CBD oil flavor that does not cause nausea, as pregnancy increases sensitivity to smell and taste.

43: RELIEVES MENSTRUAL CRAMPS

Women around the globe can commiserate in the monthly pain that is menstrual cramps. Dysmenorrhea (or painful menstruation) is common in women, and symptoms range from pelvic, stomach, and back pain, to cramping, fatigue, and headaches. Store-bought treatments like heating pads, aspirin, and caffeine work for some women, but for many, the pain is still too much—or the side effects of OTC painkillers (like stomach upset) are undesirable.

CBD oil has emerged as an effective way to reduce cramping in many parts of the body, including the uterus. The female reproductive system has a very high concentration of cannabinoid receptors that are involved in regulating fertility. Endocannabinoid levels also appear to be linked with estrogen levels. When levels of the endocannabinoid anandamide are low, women experience more symptoms of PMS and period cramping. CBD oil can boost these levels of anandamide, reduce inflammation, relax muscles, and improve mood. CBD also activates the vanilloid receptor, which can reduce the perception of pain. Taken daily as a tincture, drink, or edible, CBD oil can prevent hormonal imbalances that trigger painful periods before they start. Lotions, creams, and balms containing CBD oil can also be applied to the pelvis and back to directly relieve pain and spasms, making the monthly menstrual cycle a more comfortable experience. For best results, take 15 milligrams of CBD oil under the tongue daily during the menstrual cycle and increase to 25 milligrams 1–2 times per day while experiencing menstrual cramping.

44: PROMOTES HEALTHY SEX DRIVE

For many people, particularly women, the motivation to initiate or accept sexual activity just isn't there, no matter how hard they try. Low levels of the hormone testosterone, certain medical conditions, and commonly prescribed medications like antidepressants can all interfere with desire for sex.

CBD oil can help balance hormones and clear your mind so you are in the mood for sex. Some people are easily distracted by racing thoughts or shiny objects, and can't keep focused on initiating and following through on sexual activity. CBD activates serotonin receptors that can keep you focused and excited by sex, and ease anxiety that may be preventing you from getting in the mood. By increasing levels of oxytocin and dopamine, two hormones related to pleasure and bonding, CBD oil can also make sex feel more enjoyable, leading to your seeking it rather than avoiding it. Taking 15–25 milligrams of CBD oil daily is best for increasing your sex drive. You can also mix the CBD oil into a delicious latte that boosts its sensual effects.

TO MAKE A SENSUAL CBD TEA, GATHER:

1 bag caffeinated or caffeine-free hibiscus tea
1 bag caffeinated or caffeine-free green tea
1 bag caffeinated or caffeine-free ginger tea
1 bag caffeinated or caffeine-free chamomile tea
6 cups hot water
100 milligrams CBD oil
4 tablespoons pure honey

Steep tea in hot water for 5 minutes. Remove the tea bags, add CBD oil and honey, and stir.

RECOMMENDATIONS FOR USE

This recipe makes 4 servings. Store in the refrigerator in an airtight container for up to five days. When ready to drink, make 1 serving by adding 1½ cups tea mix to the mug. You can also add warm coconut milk. Drink 30 minutes before bedroom activity.

45: REDUCES MARIJUANA WITHDRAWAL

Some people confuse CBD oil with cannabis or its slang terms (marijuana, pot, or weed), but they are very different. Besides the fact that CBD oil does not produce the euphoric high that THC-rich cannabis does, CBD oil is nonaddictive, has few side effects, and does not cause withdrawal symptoms. Those who have smoked THC-rich cannabis every day for years will have the hardest time quitting marijuana. While less than half of marijuana smokers will ever exhibit withdrawal symptoms, the symptoms of marijuana withdrawal include the following:

▓ Anxiety, irritability, and depression.
▓ Loss of focus and boredom.
▓ Insomnia and other sleep issues.
▓ Headaches and stomach issues.
▓ Sweating and chills.
▓ Cravings for marijuana.

These withdrawal symptoms are often so intense that 78 percent of marijuana smokers who experience them smoke marijuana again to relieve them.

Fortunately, CBD oil can boost levels of the natural endocannabinoid anandamide and rebalance the brain during marijuana withdrawal. CBD oil can also promote sleep, reduce anxiety, and relax the body, making quitting marijuana smoking as comfortable as possible.

HOW TO USE

Topical CBD oil products such as lotions, creams, or bath bombs will do little to help as the CBD is not absorbed into the bloodstream and won't travel to the brain. Make sure to ingest CBD oil at a dosage of 25–30 milligrams under the tongue 3–4 times per day to successfully manage symptoms of marijuana withdrawal, as cravings or irritability will come back once the CBD oil wears off.

46: STIMULATES APPETITE IN THE UNDERWEIGHT

As much as the media focuses on weight loss, the reality is there are also many people who struggle to eat or gain weight. A number of conditions and medications come with loss of appetite, including anorexia, nausea, pregnancy, Parkinson's disease, Crohn's disease, AIDS, and chemotherapy treatment for cancer. Other times, it's simply a fast metabolism that keeps someone's weight dangerously low.

Lack of appetite is notoriously hard to treat, but CBD oil provides a natural solution. Full-spectrum CBD oil contains numerous cannabinoids like CBD and THC that stimulate the appetite by activating cannabinoid receptors in the brain regions that regulate eating. THC has also been FDA-approved to stimulate appetite in patients with cancer or HIV since 1985. Several studies have found increased hunger is a common side effect of CBD oil, especially in people who are underweight. Coconut MCT oil found in most formulations of CBD oil can help soothe an inflamed stomach, fight bacterial infections, and make eating less painful.

HOW TO USE

Choose a full-spectrum CBD oil tincture as opposed to a broad-spectrum CBD oil, which does not have THC. Also look for a CBD oil rich in the terpene myrcene, which stimulates hunger, and avoid those rich in the terpene humulene, which suppresses hunger. CBD oil may decrease appetite or cause stomach upset in some people. Discontinue CBD oil use if you are experiencing these side effects.

47: CALMS ANGER

In 2018, one in fifty-nine children in the United States were diagnosed with autism, a common neurocognitive disorder persisting into adulthood that results in disordered communication and behaviors, including outbursts of rage. A 2019 study published in the journal *Molecular Autism* found children with autism have lowered blood levels of several endocannabinoids, including anandamide. These alterations in the endocannabinoid system suggest that supplementation with CBD oil can help rebalance the brain of patients with autism, as CBD increases levels of the endocannabinoid anandamide, which bind to CB1 and CB2 receptors. CBD oil also modulates the activity of serotonin, dopamine, glutamate, and GABA receptors, repairing altered brain chemistry in autism. By activating serotonin receptors, CBD can relieve anxiety, calming rage, preventing self-harm, and promoting sleep.

Of course, irritability and rage aren't linked to just autism. They can also be symptoms of certain personality disorders, mental health conditions including bipolar disorder, and simply the stress of everyday life. Whether or not you have an official diagnosis, using 10–20 milligrams of CBD oil under the tongue can help you stay calm despite the frustrations of the day.

TAKE CARE

While most patients see reduction in rage when using CBD oil, a small percentage of patients do worse. Talk to your doctor before using CBD oil if you have been diagnosed with autism or any other serious condition.

48: MAXIMIZES MASSAGES

Massages aren't just a luxury; they are an amazing tool to lower stress, increase flexibility, alleviate pain, and boost your immune system. Monthly massages also have the ability to safely manage back, muscle, and joint pain without the need for painkillers, making them a must for anyone with chronic pain.

CBD oil applied to the skin before a massage can relax muscles, lower inflammation, boost circulation, and reduce pain. In other words, CBD massage oil will help you power through that deep tissue massage you really need but always avoid because it hurts so much. It also boosts the effects of the massage itself. You can also take 10–25 milligrams of CBD oil as a tincture before your massage session to double up on its healing and relaxation effects.

Check to see if your local massage place includes CBD lotion or CBD massage oil as an add-on. If not, simply ask if you can bring your own CBD oil for the massage therapist to apply. Massage oils purchased at the store can come with synthetic ingredients like fragrance, coloring, and preservatives that aren't safe for your skin and can give you a headache. So it's always best to make your own. Follow the recipe provided to create your own CBD massage oil in minutes.

TO MAKE A RELAXING CBD MASSAGE OIL, GATHER:

½ cup organic coconut oil

12 drops lavender essential oil

8 drops orange essential oil

150 milligrams CBD oil

Warm up coconut oil to liquid form by heating in the microwave for intervals of 30 seconds. Mix in remaining ingredients. Store at room temperature in an airtight container for up to six months.

49: HELPS LOWER RISK OF CANCER

At some point in their lifetime, four in ten Americans will develop cancer. Unfortunately, once cancer is diagnosed, often it has already grown to a decent size, or has spread to other areas in the body that may make it difficult to treat. Modern medicine focuses on treating cancer instead of preventing it, which is why it's up to us to pursue lifestyle changes that can reduce our risk of developing cancer.

CBD oil is uniquely positioned to fight the environmental risks we can't avoid that contribute to cancer risk. Endocannabinoid deficiency is linked to a variety of cancers; anandamide is reduced in breast cancer, and low levels of endocannabinoids may create an environment for cancer to thrive in. By boosting the endocannabinoid system with CBD oil, we may be able to prevent the production of deadly tumors. A more powerful antioxidant than vitamin C or vitamin E, CBD has the ability to neutralize free radicals before they damage DNA and turn cells cancerous. More specifically, CBD activates expression of the protein called Nrf2, which is the "master regulator" of the antioxidant response and turns on hundreds of genes that control everything from immune response to growth of tumors. Taking just 15 milligrams of CBD oil daily could safely raise your body's cancer defenses. Choose full-spectrum CBD oil, which contains both THC and THCA, cannabinoids that are powerful at preventing cancer. CBDA, also found in CBD oil, acts like a COX-2 inhibitor, and can help prevent skin tumors caused by overexposure to the sun or tanning beds.

50: BALANCES THE IMMUNE SYSTEM

Having a healthy immune system is the first line of defense against toxins and microbes you encounter in your home, workplace, and public spaces. From the food you eat to the restrooms you frequent, you are constantly facing objects that your body's immune system can either attack or ignore. If you have a hyperactive immune system and an autoimmune disorder, your body treats every foreign object as a danger, and even attacks the healthy tissue in your gut, skin, and other body regions in defense. On the flipside, people with sluggish immune systems are constantly coming down with colds and heal slowly as they don't fight off microbes well. While medications to increase or decrease immunity exist, many have dangerous side effects or are expensive.

CBD oil offers new hope to those who have been frustrated with their health. The endocannabinoid system provides balance to the numerous cellular systems in the body, including the immune system. If someone has a hyperactive immune system that is releasing too many cytokines and attacking its own tissue, taking CBD oil can quiet it. In fact, patients with lupus, psoriasis, and other autoimmune disorders report decreased inflammation after using CBD oil. On the flip side, phytocannabinoids in CBD oil can directly kill some types of viruses and bacteria, as well as stimulate the immune system to attack them in those experiencing a depressed immune system (which can stem from poor diet, drug and alcohol use, and certain medications and medical conditions). Whether or not you need to boost your immune system or slow it down, taking 10–25 milligrams of CBD oil each day can balance your body's immune response and protect it from cellular damage.

51: INCREASES ANTIBACTERIAL ACTIVITY

Protecting the body from bacteria is crucial to good health, as once they enter the body, they are attacked by the immune system, causing inflammation. Bacteria on the skin and mucous membranes can cause infections, and bacteria eaten in food can cause nausea, vomiting, diarrhea, and even damage to the lining of the gut. While proper cooking and hygiene, including hand washing and tooth brushing, can prevent most bacterial infections, many people slip up from time to time and get sick. Some reach for synthetic antibacterial products like counter sprays and hand gels but overuse of these products and of antibiotics has led to bacteria becoming resistant. A healthier way to prevent exposure to bacteria is by using natural products like CBD oil.

CBD oil contains terpenes and phytocannabinoids that powerfully fight off bacteria. A study published in the *Journal of Natural Products* found that, when CBD is used in conjunction with antibiotics, it increases their antibacterial activity. This suggests CBD oil may be a way to fight bacterial infections whether they are present in skin wounds or internal. Humulene and limonene are two terpenes in CBD oil that kill bacteria. Additionally, CBD, CBG, CBC, CBN, and THC, potent phytocannabinoids in full-spectrum CBD oil, have been found to be active against a strain of antibiotic resistant staph bacteria, called a MRSA infection. CBG and CBD in particular appear to have the most robust activity against MRSA. For the best results, take 10–25 milligrams of CBD oil daily to protect against exposure to bacteria, and increase to 25–50 milligrams of CBD oil if you have an active infection.

52: HELPS RELEASE PAINFUL MEMORIES

An area of the brain called the hippocampus is responsible for learning and memory, and is rich in cannabinoid receptors. Activating these cannabinoid receptors doesn't help you learn; in fact, it helps you forget. While too much forgetfulness can be harmful, forgetting some things like painful memories of breakups, violence, or other trauma can be beneficial to your overall health and happiness. When we can't let go, our brain replays those memories over and over again during the day as flashbacks and at night as nightmares. Some people who experience trauma develop post-traumatic stress disorder (PTSD), which has symptoms of anxiety, hypervigilance, aggression, and insomnia that can last for decades. Several studies looking at the level of endocannabinoids in the blood of patients who have experienced trauma have found they have an endocannabinoid deficiency.

Veterans and other groups who are at high risk for PTSD often use cannabis or CBD oil to find relief. Because CBD oil contains multiple phytocannabinoids that restore balance to the endocannabinoid system, it helps them think less about their traumas. Several clinical trials have investigated the use of CBD and THC for PTSD, and all have had positive results. In order to benefit from CBD oil in this case, you must eat it rather than use it topically, because topicals won't get into your bloodstream. Taking 25–50 milligrams of full-spectrum CBD oil daily is recommended, as THC helps the CBD be more effective at suppressing unwanted memories.

53: EASES BREATHING

Asthma is a common but potentially deadly lung condition that more than twenty-five million Americans suffer from. Coughing, wheezing, chest tightness, and shortness of breath are hallmarks of the condition; allergies, pollution, cigarette smoke, stress, and living in a city can all trigger an asthma attack. Some people have life-threatening asthma attacks and have to limit physical activity; others are barely bothered by their asthma. While there are many medications available for people with asthma, the options are not great. Traditional treatments for acute asthma attacks include inhalers with stimulants that can trigger anxiety, making an asthma attack worse, and oral medications that have many unpleasant side effects.

A natural remedy, CBD oil can improve the efficacy of traditional asthma treatments and reduce the impact of side effects. This CBD oil–infused cocktail recipe is perfect for relaxing anywhere without breathing issues, thanks to the health benefits of these ingredients:

- CBD oil: Relaxes airways, both preventing asthma and lessening attacks.

- Rosemary: Contains high levels of pinene, a terpene that opens airways.
- Ginger: Reduces inflammation throughout the body.
- Vodka: Relieves stress and increases blood flow.

TO MAKE A ROSEMARY BREEZE COCKTAIL, GATHER:

1 small sprig fresh rosemary

4 slices fresh ginger, grated

1 tablespoon lemon juice

10 milligrams CBD oil

Ice to fill glass

2 ounces organic vodka

½ cup ginger ale

Muddle rosemary and ginger in lemon juice in an old-fashioned glass. Add CBD oil, stir, and add ice. Add vodka and then ginger ale. Enjoy immediately.

54: REDUCES RISK OF HEART ATTACK

A heart attack is a common but terrifying experience, occurring when one of the arteries in your heart is blocked, blood flow is stopped, and the heart muscle is deprived of nutrients and oxygen. Every year, over one million Americans will have a heart attack, and 14 percent will die from it. Heart attack is most likely to occur in the thirty million Americans diagnosed with heart disease. Men over forty-five years of age and women over the age of fifty-five are more likely than younger people to have a heart attack, but it can happen at any age. While some risk factors like a family history of having heart attacks or an autoimmune disorder like lupus cannot be changed, many others are in your control. You can reduce your risk of heart attack at any age by quitting smoking, decreasing the amount of bad cholesterol in your diet, exercising regularly, avoiding stimulants such as cocaine or Adderall, managing your response to stress, and, yes, by taking CBD oil.

A wellness dose of CBD oil tincture of between 10–25 milligrams taken daily helps keep your heart healthy. CBD directly activates a type of serotonin receptor called 5-HT1A, which can relieve anxiety and further reduce stress on the heart. CBD oil is also full of antioxidants and anti-inflammatories that can promote heart health and prevent cardiovascular disease by doing the following:

- Increasing blood flow through arteries.
- Lowering blood pressure.
- Maintaining regular heart beats.

TAKE CARE

If you have serious cardiac issues, avoid using full-spectrum CBD oil containing THC, as THC may exacerbate heart arrhythmias in some patients. Talk to your doctor before starting a daily regimen of CBD oil.

55: SLOWS ALS PROGRESSION

One of the most devastating neurological diseases, amyotrophic lateral sclerosis (ALS) causes brain cells that control movement to get damaged and die, preventing most types of voluntary and involuntary movement. ALS (or Lou Gehrig's disease) is more common than some might suspect, with 450,000 worldwide living with this incurable disease. Because this disease often comes on with no warning and symptoms accelerate rapidly, treatments do little to slow the disease and mostly offer only comfort. Symptoms of ALS include muscle weakness, twitching, and cramping; inability to walk, speak, and breathe without support; and cognitive issues like uncontrollable laughter or crying.

CBD oil has emerged as a natural treatment to improve the quality of life in patients with ALS, as well as a potential neuroprotectant. CBD oil contains numerous antioxidants and anti-inflammatories that protect brain cells from damage and death caused by free radicals. While a clinical trial in Australia is investigating whether CBD oil actually slows the progression of ALS, patients are already using CBD oil both topically and orally to boost their physical and emotional health.

Phytocannabinoids in full-spectrum CBD oil, including CBD and THC, can help relieve muscle spasms, improve mood, reduce pain, promote sleep, and keep up the appetite in many people with the disease.

TAKE CARE

Dosing for patients with neurodegenerative conditions like ALS is much different than wellness doses for healthy people, and it is not effective for all patients. Doses of CBD oil that protect the brain can range from 50–200 milligrams and more per day; you should always talk to your physician before starting a daily regimen of CBD oil.

56: EASES PAIN FROM ENDOMETRIOSIS

Worldwide, 176 million women suffer from endometriosis, a condition where endometrial tissue grows outside the uterus, where it may also cause bleeding. Inflammation, pelvic pain, and cramping outside of the menstrual cycle, as well as nausea and vomiting, headaches, back pain, and gastrointestinal issues are all common in patients with endometriosis. Symptoms can range from mild to so completely debilitating that it prevents women from working, going to school, or taking care of the family. Treatments focus on palliative care rather than treating the root cause of the problem, and include multiple surgeries to remove tissue, medications that shut down monthly menstrual cycles, opioid painkillers, antidepressants, and steroid anti-inflammatories. Many of these treatments are expensive, have dangerous side effects (including risk of addiction, blood clots, or even death), and are ineffective at managing symptoms. Women are now turning to natural remedies like CBD oil for a healthier alternative to improve the quality of their lives with this painful condition.

CBD oil contains phytocannabinoids that activate cannabinoid receptors that are abundant in the uterus, ovaries, and other reproductive tissues. One theory of endometriosis is that a dysfunction of the endocannabinoid system is the root cause, and by restoring balance to this system through CBD oil, hormonal issues and disease symptoms are resolved. CBD and THC have been used in animal trials to stop the migration of endometriosis tissue, and patients using CBD oil have found symptom relief. CBD oil can reduce inflammation, relieve pain, and stop cramping. CBD oil also contains terpenes and phytocannabinoids that improve mood and even boost serotonin, helping with the nausea and vomiting that come with the chronic pain from endometriosis. Taking 15–25 milligrams of CBD oil twice daily can make living with endometriosis more comfortable.

57: FIGHTS INFLAMMATION

When white blood cells attack foreign microbes, releasing antibodies and inflammatory cytokines, it causes tissue to be inflamed. Inflammation can occur anywhere in your body, from your colon to your eyes. While inflammation can be a healthy response to an acute injury or stressor, chronic inflammation is thought to be the root cause of many diseases, including heart disease and cancer. It's possible to have chronic inflammation throughout your body and not be aware of it, as the standard American diet (SAD) is full of toxins and fats that keep us feeling sluggish, unwell, and aching all over. Inflammation can cause numerous health issues, including pain and tissue damage; but the medications people take to treat it can also have serious side effects, including liver damage. Anti-inflammatory medications range from over-the-counter NSAIDs to strong steroids, yet many people who take them long term find they become less effective at controlling their inflammation. To truly heal the body, it takes changing the diet and adding healthy supplements like CBD oil to the mix.

The chemical compounds in full-spectrum and broad-spectrum CBD oil, including phytocannabinoids, terpenes, flavonoids, and fatty acids, all heal tissue damaged by inflammation. CBD, THC, and other cannabinoids in CBD oil activate CB2 receptors on immune cells to quiet them. Beta-caryophyllene, linalool, myrcene, pinene, and humulene are all terpenes in CBD oil that reduce the release of inflammatory compounds. The flavonoids quercetin and apigenin that are abundant in CBD oil further suppress inflammation. The most common carrier oil used in CBD oil, MCT oil, contains high levels of capric acid, which has potent anti-inflammatory properties. To stay active in the fight against inflammation, take 10–25 milligrams of CBD oil daily.

58: INCREASES BLOOD FLOW TO THE BRAIN

The brain is the most important organ in the human body, yet so many of us aren't doing everything we can to keep it fueled and in top shape. Sixty percent of all the glucose in the body is used by the brain, requiring rapid circulation of blood through the body. When blood flow is slowed or blocked, the brain suffers. Stimulants like caffeine, cigarettes, and cocaine are vasoconstrictors, which are substances that can increase the risk of blood clots and stroke. CBD oil contains phytocannabinoids like CBD and THC that are vasodilators, substances that widen blood vessels and lower blood pressure. This increases blood flow to the brain, enhancing the flow of critical nutrients, including oxygen, to the brain. Enhanced blood flow also works to flush away cellular debris and toxins.

CBD oil also has profound neuroprotective effects, as verified by US Patent 6,630,507. A research study by Fukuoka University found that CBD can reduce brain damage from a stroke. This means phytocannabinoids in CBD oil activate serotonin receptors to cause release of nitric oxide in blood vessels and improve blood flow. It's possible that using 15–25 milligrams of CBD oil daily could keep the brain healthy so that it can bounce back more easily from injury or stroke. Taking CBD oil after a stroke has already occurred can also speed brain repair. Brain damage from stroke causes free radical damage, inflammation, and blood clots, all of which the antioxidants and anti-inflammatories in CBD oil fight. Taking CBD oil as you age could be key to protecting your brain.

TAKE CARE

CBD oil may interact with drugs prescribed for stroke, including blood thinners. Talk to your doctor before taking CBD oil.

59: SOOTHES MOTION SICKNESS

Motion sickness is the feeling of nausea when riding in a moving object such as a boat, car, train, or airplane. Some people never experience it at all, while others experience mild to severe symptoms. Patients that suffer from frequent nausea, migraines, or insomnia may be more likely to have motion sickness. Women are more susceptible to having motion sickness, and pregnancy, menstruation, and the use of hormonal birth control increases the risk of experiencing it. Drug and alcohol use can also exacerbate motion sickness.

An imbalance in the endocannabinoid system can cause motion sickness or make it worse. A commonly prescribed medication for motion sickness, dexamethasone, works by increasing levels of endocannabinoids, including anandamide, and activating cannabinoid receptors in the brain and stomach. CBD oil can increase levels of anandamide, restoring balance to the endocannabinoid system. CBD oil can also reduce symptoms of nausea and vomiting, eliminating motion sickness symptoms fast. It is always easier to prevent motion sickness than it is to treat it, so before going on a cruise or other trip where you know you might experience motion sickness, remember to take or increase your daily dose of CBD oil. Use the following recipe for a refreshing CBD oil tonic you can sip to combat motion sickness. Use a citrus-flavored CBD oil for the best results.

TO MAKE A CBD OIL TONIC, GATHER:

1 cup ginger ale
25 milligrams CBD oil
1 cup ice cubes

Combine all ingredients and drink. After consuming the drink, eat one slice fresh or candied ginger to further help with nausea. Drink up to 3 times daily to minimize motion sickness.

TAKE CARE

Taking CBD oil with OTC medications for motion sickness may result in increased dizziness, drowsiness, or confusion. Use only natural remedies with CBD oil.

60: ENCOURAGES HEALTHY LIVER FUNCTION

A healthy liver is key to detoxifying the blood, removing toxic chemicals, and breaking down drugs. When the liver is damaged by heavy drinking, cancer, medical conditions, or poor diet, it fails to function properly, and can wreak havoc on the body. A sick liver causes buildup of toxins in the body, leading to free radical damage to cells and chronic illness.

CBD oil can protect the liver against damage, fight infections, and even repair liver damage. Antioxidants in CBD oil protect against toxic heavy metals acting as free radicals that can mutate or kill liver cells. CBD oil contains numerous anti-inflammatories that directly fight liver inflammation, but it also works in a unique way by activating the endocannabinoid system to suppress an overactive immune system. CBD activates CB2 receptors that kill white blood cells attacking liver cells in autoimmune hepatitis. If the source of liver inflammation is viral, whether due to the flu or hepatitis, phytocannabinoids in CBD oil are potent antivirals and have been the focus of numerous research studies.

Everyone has accumulated liver damage from a lifetime of exposure to toxins in food, drugs, alcohol, and infections. By starting a healthy diet, avoiding synthetic chemicals, and taking a dose of 10–25 milligrams of CBD oil each day, you can allow damaged liver tissue to heal. CBD oil can be your key to unlocking a healthier body.

61: EASES SYMPTOMS OF PARKINSON'S DISEASE

More than ten million people worldwide are living with Parkinson's, a disease with no known cause or cure, that leaves patients struggling to do simple tasks and often needing home care. Symptoms of Parkinson's disease include the following:

■ Tremors in the hands and fingers.
■ Slow movement and problems walking.
■ Impaired sense of balance.
■ Poor posture, including hunched back.
■ Rigid, painful muscles.
■ Slurred or soft speech.
■ Inability to write by hand.
■ Mood changes, including depression.
■ Cognitive impairment, including memory loss.
■ Sleep issues, including insomnia.

Preventing further destruction of dopamine neurons in the brain and increasing dopamine release are keys to treating Parkinson's disease. Many patients with Parkinson's are not responsive to traditional medications, and their symptoms get worse with age.

While CBD oil is not a cure for Parkinson's disease, its unique ability to balance brain neurotransmitters as well as offset the side effects of medications are essential to improving quality of life in patients with the disease. CBD oil contains antioxidants and anti-inflammatories that can protect dopamine cells from dying, delaying progression of the disease. Cannabinoids in CBD oil help relax rigid muscles, slow tremors, and increase appetite, while its terpenes such as pinene can fight brain fog and improve focus. Finally, the most common carrier oil used in CBD oil, coconut MCT oil, is helpful for easing the constipation that patients with Parkinson's disease experience.

HOW TO USE

20 milligrams of CBD oil taken as a tincture 3 times a day is optimal to improve mood, sleep, and motor function in patients with Parkinson's disease. Applying CBD oil topically is not likely to be effective, as the source of dysfunction is in the brain, not the muscle.

62: ENHANCES STRESS RELIEF FROM YOGA

Yoga's combination of exercise and mindfulness makes it a killer stress reliever. Yoga has been practiced for thousands of years as a way to relax the mind and keep the body fit. In fact, clinical studies have shown practicing yoga for as little as 1–2 sessions a week can lower levels of the stress hormone cortisol and reduce symptoms of depression. Whether you call it ganja yoga, cannabis yoga, or CBD yoga, more and more yoga teachers are training their students on the proper use and health benefits of taking CBD oil before and after a yoga workout. Unlike THC-rich cannabis, CBD oil will not get you high. Taking 15–25 milligrams of CBD oil as a tincture or drinking it 10 minutes before yoga can help relieve any anxiety you have, making it easier to get out of your head and de-stress in your session. Phytocannabinoids in CBD oil can help ease muscle tension and stiffness, increasing your flexibility and helping you hold yoga poses longer. Terpenes in CBD oil like pinene may help open up airways, allowing you to breathe in more deeply, oxygenating your muscles and exhaling all your stress.

After a vigorous yoga session, apply CBD oil lotions and creams to your neck, back, legs, or arms to relieve muscle pain, inflammation, and soreness. With less pain, yoga will be more pleasurable, and you won't have to wait to recover before your next workout. By combining CBD oil as a tincture before yoga and as a topical after yoga, you'll be able to accelerate your emotional and physical healing.

63: REDUCES FEARS AND PHOBIAS

From spiders to heights to clowns, everyone is afraid of something. While some fears have a basis in survival (like avoiding deadly spider bites), others are triggered by traumatic experiences or an escalation of anxiety disorders that turn into phobias (such as an irrational intolerance or aversion to an object). Phobias are actually quite common, with over 11 percent of Americans experiencing them at some point in their lifetime. When people are triggered by their phobia, they experience symptoms similar to a panic attack such as fear, dizziness, increased heart rate, inability to breathe, nausea, or dissociation. Most people don't seek treatment for their phobia, but the ones who do may require medication or exposure therapy to manage their symptoms. Because treatment can be expensive or have unwanted side effects, natural remedies for phobias are a great alternative.

The terpenes and cannabinoids in CBD oil provide an inexpensive way to reduce your stress response so that you're less likely to be triggered by unexpected exposure to your fear (and if you are triggered, more likely to experience milder symptoms). CBD oil increases serotonin, dopamine, and endocannabinoid system activity, rebalancing your brain chemistry. For people with social phobias, CBD oil can boost oxytocin levels, which may make social interactions more pleasurable. Taking just 15–30 milligrams of CBD oil a day could help you relax your mind and feel calmer around people, places, and things that usually stress you out.

64: STIMULATES BONE GROWTH

After the age of forty, we slowly start losing bone mass, and our bones become less strong and more likely to break. We even shrink 1–2 inches in height by age seventy! Postmenopausal women have a greater risk of losing bone mass than men and younger women. Other risk factors for bone loss and osteoporosis include smoking, heavy drinking, long-term steroid medication use, low body height and weight, and family history.

Breaking a bone is a painful ordeal, whether it's from an accident or from a disease like osteoporosis, which affects 30 percent of postmenopausal Caucasian women. Recovery can be slow, it can disrupt your ability to work or take care of your family, and your bone might not heal completely. To build strong bones, it's important to consume vitamins and minerals that strengthen them. Thankfully, full-spectrum or broad-spectrum CBD oil contains minerals such as calcium, manganese, and magnesium that do just that.

The endocannabinoid system regulates bone growth and remodeling. Activating CB1 receptors on nerves on skeletal muscle can help build bone; activating CB2 receptors on bone cells stops the age-related destruction of bone tissue. The numerous phytocannabinoids in CBD oil that stimulate bone growth include CBD, CBDV, CBN, THC, and THCV. CBD itself has been shown to boost the healing of bone fractures. Taking CBD oil daily can be a great natural way to build bone, prevent age-related bone loss, and heal broken bones.

65: SUPPORTS A LONGER LIFE SPAN

While the average American lives for seventy-eight years, this life span is lower than that of other industrialized countries due to the unhealthy standard American diet, lack of exercise, chronic stress, sleep deprivation, and other lifestyle factors. One of the main reasons why the body ages is the shortening of DNA in our cells. Telomeres, which protect the ends of our strands of DNA, get shorter each time our cells divide. After some point, the telomeres are too short to protect the DNA, and the DNA damage causes the cell to die. This process of cellular aging is called senescence.

One of the most powerful but little-known secrets of CBD oil is the number of compounds in it that protect telomeres, repair DNA damage, and ultimately help slow aging. CBD oil can reduce oxidative stress and inflammation in the body, which reduces the amount of DNA damage in the body. CBD oil is also rich in multiple types of flavonoids that are usually only found in vegetables like broccoli and soybeans. These flavonoids, including quercetin, fisetin, genistein, apigenin, and kaempferol, are well researched and potent extenders of life span. Along with CBD, these flavonoids activate a protein called Nrf2 which turns on thousands of genes that regulate our antioxidant response and promote healthy aging. By taking just 10–25 milligrams of CBD oil a day, you can activate this pathway to turn on anticancer genes and turn off procancer genes, keep your cells free of mutations, and help your body live a long and healthy life.

66: PROMOTES HEALTHY VAGINAL LUBRICATION

Vaginal dryness occurs when levels of the hormone estrogen drop, reducing vaginal lubrication and flexibility. There are many reasons for this drop in estrogen that results in vaginal dryness, including chronic stress, medical conditions (including depression), medications (including chemotherapy), breastfeeding, cigarette smoking, and menopause. Treatments like hormone replacement therapy (HRT) can be dangerous, with side effects that impact heart health. Water-based lubricants can be messy and expose you to synthetic chemicals that aren't absorbed by the sensitive mucous membranes of the vagina. Homemade natural remedies like CBD oil topicals can heal vaginal tissue, restoring some of its lubrication and suppleness.

When CBD oil is applied directly to vaginal tissue, its phytocannabinoids activate the high number of cannabinoid receptors there. This stimulates blood flow and lubrication, while reducing unpleasant inflammation and dryness. Comically referred to in the media as the "weed tampon," CBD oil suppositories are one of the best ways to continuously coat the vagina with CBD oil while you sleep, increasing the likelihood that its effects will last for days.

TO MAKE MOISTURIZING CBD VAGINAL SUPPOSITORIES, GATHER:

1½ cups organic coconut oil

10 drops lavender essential oil

10 drops frankincense essential oil

10 drops tea tree essential oil

500 milligrams CBD oil

Combine ingredients together. Using a dropper, transfer mixture to suppository molds. Let harden overnight in the freezer before using.

RECOMMENDATIONS FOR USE

Store in foil and place in the freezer for up to six months. Insert the suppository with your finger or a plastic applicator as far up the vagina as is comfortable. Use 1–3 times a week as needed (preferably at bedtime to prevent leakage).

67: LESSENS AGING OF THE BRAIN

Boosting your brain's ability to learn, remember, and process complex decisions shifts from a want to a need as you get closer to the retirement years and beyond. Levels of antioxidants and neurotransmitters become depleted the older we get, and our cognitive function slows. We can no longer bounce back from chronic stress, poor diet, lack of sleep, a couple of alcoholic drinks, or exposure to toxic chemicals. Our brains become inflamed as we age, and our ability to clear cellular garbage from our brains is greatly reduced. In some people with genetic risk for Alzheimer's, Huntington's, or Parkinson's disease, abnormal proteins can accumulate in the brain and cause neurodegeneration beyond normal aging.

Whether your brain is healthy or facing rapid aging, natural supplements like CBD oil can help you stay sharp in your later years. CBD oil can protect the brain from further injury, reduce inflammation, improve memory, and boost brain function overall. In 2003, the United States government patented cannabinoids in CBD oil for their use as antioxidants and neuroprotectants in patent 6,630,507. Even though there is still ambiguity surrounding the idea of adult neurogenesis, CBD oil can stimulate the birth of new brain cells in the hippocampus, the learning and memory center of the brain. These new brain cells keep the brain young and flexible. Unlike THC-rich cannabis, which can harm memory, CBD oil promotes better memory. Out of all the terpenes in CBD oil, pinene is renowned for promoting focus, alertness, and even improving short-term memory. By activating CB2 receptors in the brain, CBD oil also improves blood flow, increasing delivery of nutrients and accelerating the removal of toxic cellular waste that could damage cells. Taking 15–30 milligrams of CBD oil each day can help you and your brain age gracefully.

68: ALLEVIATES ALTITUDE SICKNESS

Breathing is crucial to life, but it's not always easy if you ski or hike in the largest mountains around the world. Each year, many casual travelers are unprepared for the physical requirements of breathing air with less oxygen at higher altitudes. For every 1,000 feet of elevation over 5,000 feet (or 1 mile) above sea level, it becomes exponentially harder to breathe, and symptoms like headaches, nausea, vomiting, and breathlessness can occur for up to a week until you are acclimated to the elevation. When you permanently move to a location at high altitude, your brain chemistry actually shifts; less serotonin and more dopamine is produced at a mile high, and some people experience long-term symptoms like depressed mood. Many people are not aware of the reason why they feel lethargic and unmotivated, and do nothing about it. Others tell their doctor, and are prescribed antidepressants that have undesirable side effects like nausea, headaches, and sexual dysfunction.

The hundreds of plant compounds in CBD oil all synergize to help balance brain chemistry and accelerate adaptation to elevation. Phytocannabinoid CBD boosts serotonin release and directly activates serotonin receptors, fighting headaches, nausea, fatigue, and depression. Other cannabinoids present in trace amounts in full-spectrum CBD oil, including THC and CBN, can powerfully increase appetite, which can improve energy levels and get you moving. Terpenes in CBD oil can also improve sleep quality, which will help you feel more rested in the morning and fight the fatigue from breathing in less oxygen. To beat acute altitude sickness, start taking 25 milligrams of CBD oil the day before heading to a higher elevation and continue using daily for one week. To balance the brain for a permanent move to an elevation of 1 mile or higher, take 15 milligrams of CBD oil daily for as long as you live there.

69: NURTURES BALANCED MOODS

The increasing demands and stress of contemporary life have led to a greater incidence of people who suffer from mood disorders such as depression and bipolar disorder, and from psychoses such as schizophrenia. While mental health disorders are very common (over 10 percent of Americans experience one each year), diagnosis and treatment is lacking. Therapy and prescription medications for mood disorders are expensive and often not covered by health insurance. Sadly, low-income people who lack health insurance are more likely to have mood disorders yet are not able to get diagnosed or treated. Whether or not you can afford professional treatment, you can reach for natural remedies to help stabilize your moods and make life less painful and more pleasurable.

Stress boosts the release of the hormone cortisol, which exacerbates chemical imbalances in the brain and the symptoms of mood disorders. The phytocannabinoids in CBD oil have the unique ability to balance brain chemistry, bringing your mood down if you are feeling manic, or lifting you up if you are feeling depressed. Because CBD oil can directly activate serotonin receptors, it can work to relieve anxiety and help ground you in reality.

HOW TO USE

Clinical trials have shown that CBD oil is effective at treating schizophrenia and bipolar disorder, but treatment requires taking doses much higher than the average. To be safe, take no more than 25–50 milligrams of CBD oil daily and, more importantly, talk to your doctor if you are on any psychiatric medications before using CBD oil.

70: IMPROVES JOINT MOBILITY

The knee, elbow, hip, and shoulder are all examples of the connections between two or more bones or joints. Because joints undergo a lifetime of use and abuse from walking, playing sports, and many more activities, they can be easily damaged by injury and diseases like arthritis and scoliosis. When joints are damaged, they become inflamed, stiff, and painful, leading to reduced range of motion. NSAIDs such as naproxen or aspirin are the first line of treatment of damaged joints; severe cases of joint pain require prescription drugs or even surgery, which can be expensive and have unwanted side effects or long recovery times. In the worst cases, treatments actually cause more pain in the long run.

Natural treatments like CBD oil can provide relief without the expense of physical therapy or surgery while improving your overall health. Just one dose of 15–30 milligrams per day as a tincture or in food can relieve painful, inflamed joints.

This recipe contains ingredients that all work together to do the following:

- Fight inflammation.
- Lubricate joints.
- Reduce joint swelling.
- Relieve pain.
- Improve circulation.
- Enhance flexibility.

TO MAKE VEGAN GINGER ICE CREAM, GATHER:

2 medium ripe avocados, peeled and pitted
1 (13.5-ounce) can coconut milk
2 tablespoons lemon juice
1 large ripe banana
2 teaspoons pure honey
1 cup candied ginger
60 milligrams CBD oil

Blend until smooth. Transfer into a cold metal pan and freeze for 4 hours.

RECOMMENDATIONS FOR USE

Transfer ice cream to an airtight container and store for up to one month. Makes 6 servings.

71: QUIETS OVERACTIVE THOUGHTS

Having racing, obsessive, and even compulsive thoughts is more common than you might think in these stressful times. While 2.2 million Americans have an official diagnosis of obsessive-compulsive disorder (OCD), many more struggle to shut off their inner monologue and relax. Obsessive thoughts come in the form of constant worrying, avoiding germs, looking for exits, suspecting your partner is cheating on you, and more. Pharmaceutical treatments such as antidepressants and benzodiazepines come with such unpleasant side effects as addiction, nausea, headaches, and sexual dysfunction. Of the many natural remedies that people have tried, CBD oil stands out as a superior treatment.

CBD oil contains numerous phytocannabinoids and terpenes that can help boost mood and relax the mind. The terpenes linalool and myrcene relieve anxiety and promote calm, which can help you enjoy the moment instead of focusing on details that you can't control. The phytocannabinoid CBD works to balance your brain by directly activating serotonin receptors and a small subset of dopamine receptors, reducing ruminating thoughts and allowing your mind to quiet. In fact, a 2011 study by the *Journal of Psychopharmacology* found that 400-milligram CBD oil capsules were effective at reducing obsessive-compulsive behavior. While CBD oil may help healthy people relax at wellness doses of 25–50 milligrams per day, it is an addition to, not a replacement for your current treatment regimen.

TAKE CARE

CBD oil may interact with certain psychiatric medications. Do not use it before speaking with your doctor.

72: BOOSTS FERTILITY

Millions of American women struggle with trying to become and stay pregnant. The process of growing a family can be incredibly stressful, and the inability to conceive can be caused by infertility in either partner. Some forms of infertility (such as those caused by genetics, medications, or early menopause) may be incurable, but for infertility cases where pregnancy is possible, the following are some factors affecting fertility that can be remedied:

- Anxiety about the inability to conceive.
- Stressors, including work or family.
- Hormone imbalances in either parent.
- Consuming drugs that damage the DNA of the sperm or egg.

By taking CBD oil as a daily ritual, you can mitigate these risk factors for infertility. CBD oil can help relax couples, and studies have shown that reducing stress can increase the likelihood of conceiving, whether naturally or through in vitro fertilization (IVF). Chronic inflammation can disrupt ovulation, as well as implantation of the egg in the uterus; using CBD oil as an anti-inflammatory may help normalize ovulation and boost fertility. While no studies have looked directly at how CBD oil impacts fertility, research has found that couples in which one or both partners use cannabis containing THC have no issues with conceiving. In addition, CBD oil acts as a potent antioxidant, suggesting it should protect egg and sperm cells from free-radical damage, possibly improving fertility.

PART 2

BEAUTY

Everywhere you turn, new beauty products are cropping up, promising anything from silky soft hair to skin that makes you look years younger. Unfortunately, each of these treatments targets just one part of your daily regime, and their costs add up faster than the bottles, jars, and tubes themselves. Most commercial products also contain dozens of chemicals that can lead to such unpleasant side effects as dry skin and breakouts. CBD oil can add mighty phytocannabinoids, powerful antioxidants, and essential nutrients to your skin, hair, nails, and more naturally, without breaking the bank. CBD oil activates receptors in the skin that turn on genes promoting healing and diminishing signs of aging. It is also anti-inflammatory, reducing swelling and redness. When taken as a tincture, CBD oil targets bacteria that lead to bad breath, while CBD oil conditioner boosts hair growth.

The following part offers easy recipes and tips for using CBD oil to beat blemishes, strengthen teeth, reduce wrinkles, and so much more. CBD oil may just become your favorite secret weapon in looking—and ultimately feeling—your best.

73: REDUCES ACNE

Acne is caused by oil, dirt, and bacteria building up under the skin. When skin can't shed properly, it can trap this debris, causing an infection that results in a pimple or cyst. Over 85 percent of young adults have some form of acne, with up to 30 percent seeking medical treatment for it. Many adults continue to struggle with acne if they had it as teenagers, while some get it for the first time later in life. Most acne sufferers reach toward harsh OTC and prescription topical treatments for acne that burn and dry out the skin, causing new skin problems.

CBD oil provides a natural alternative to synthetic treatments for acne. CBD oil products applied to the skin reduce oil production in the skin, keeping pores clear. CBD oil is also antibacterial, killing the bacteria that cause acne. CBD reduces inflammation, minimizing redness and pimple size when acne does occur. CBD oil works best for acne when used as both a topical treatment and ingested. Be careful, as not all products that are meant to be applied to the skin are safe to eat and vice versa. To play it safe, buy one product for skin and one product to be eaten. If you are purchasing topical CBD oil products for children, remember they aren't absorbed into the bloodstream and can be used safely by teens. The following is a simple, safe, and inexpensive acne mask that you can make in your own home.

TO MAKE A HOMEMADE ACNE MASK, COMBINE:

25 milligrams unflavored CBD oil
1 teaspoon pure honey
1 teaspoon apple cider vinegar
2 teaspoons bentonite clay

RECOMMENDATIONS FOR USE

Apply to skin immediately after combining ingredients. Wait 10 minutes for the mask to dry, then gently remove with a washcloth and warm water. Use 1–2 times per week.

74: FIGHTS SKIN AGING

As we age, the collagen in our skin breaks down, revealing fine lines and wrinkles on our face, neck, and chest. Free radicals generated from smoking cigarettes, drinking alcohol, being exposed to pollution, and eating an unhealthy diet break down collagen further, aging the skin dramatically. Many turn to expensive treatments such as lasers, injections, and prescriptions, rather than choosing preventative measures and holistic treatments. Looking to natural wrinkle treatments will save you money and protect you from the dangerous side effects of botched clinical treatments, including paralysis of the face, chemical burns, and even death.

Phytocannabinoids in CBD oil can naturally boost production of collagen, helping to plump the skin, fill in those lines, and even reduce the likelihood of new wrinkles appearing in the future. Of course, with so many ways to use CBD oil, it may seem difficult to know which products to use. Wrinkle serums are superior to wrinkle lotions and creams because the ingredients in serums are concentrated, delivering the most potent ingredients straight to where they are needed without wasting a drop. The following CBD oil serum can be applied directly to wrinkles and is safe for even acne-prone skin.

TO MAKE A CBD OIL WRINKLE SERUM, COMBINE:

2 teaspoons rosehip seed oil

1 teaspoon vitamin E oil

4 drops frankincense essential oil

25 milligrams CBD oil

RECOMMENDATIONS FOR USE

Add serum to a small roll-on applicator and store at room temperature for up to one year. Shake well before each use and apply directly to areas with wrinkles. Tap lightly into skin to enhance absorption.

75: MOISTURIZES SKIN

Your skin can go from glowing to dry and flaky within hours, depending on what you drink, where you go, and more. In fact, while drinking enough water is the number one determinant of how hydrated your skin is, wind, pollution, dry air, flying, and even stress can dry out your skin. When choosing a moisturizer for your skin or body, it's important to remember that the skin is your largest organ and can absorb both good and bad compounds into your bloodstream. Many store-bought moisturizers contain synthetic chemicals and sunscreens that can be harmful to your health, which is why you should use only natural ingredients in any skincare routine.

The endocannabinoid system has emerged as a new target for improving the appearance and health of skin. Endocannabinoids, including anandamide and 2-AG, are found in oil glands, and cannabinoid receptors are found in multiple types of cells in the skin. Applying CBD oil to the skin can boost activity of the endocannabinoid system and promote beautiful-looking skin. CBD oil is full of fatty acids, antioxidants, and anti-inflammatories that nourish the skin. No matter which carrier oil is used, CBD oil lotions, creams, and balms are full of omega-3 and omega-6 fatty acids that coat the skin and act as a barrier against wind, pollution, and irritating fabrics. Antioxidants found in CBD oil, including cannabinoids, flavonoids, and terpenes, protect skin against free radical production and sun damage, which stops skin peeling and dryness.

HOW TO USE

Apply CBD oil moisturizer generously to skin daily or as needed. Avoid CBD topical oils made for pain, as they often contain ingredients such as menthol that can dry out the skin.

76: EASES ECZEMA

More than eighteen million Americans have eczema, a red, itchy rash that appears on the arms, legs, and cheeks. Clinically known as atopic dermatitis, eczema is often a genetic condition, meaning it is passed on in families and starts in early childhood. Because eczema is caused by inflammation, it is treatable by decreasing exposure to foods and chemicals that cause irritation. Natural remedies are ideal for treating eczema, as prescription treatments have side effects that outweigh their benefits.

One botanical treatment for eczema is CBD oil, which can be taken orally to decrease inflammation throughout the body, or applied directly to the skin as a lotion, cream, or balm.

Several clinical studies have looked at the effectiveness of using topical CBD oil treatments on eczema and similar skin conditions. A 2019 study found that using CBD lotion twice a day for three weeks is a safe and effective treatment for eczema, with no allergic reactions or side effects. Besides containing powerful anti-inflammatories, CBD oil also contains phytocannabinoids that can heal the skin by activating cannabinoid receptors like CB2 and TRPV4. CBD increases levels of the endocannabinoid anandamide when applied to the skin. One study published in *Clinical Interventions in Aging* found that applying anandamide to the skin for two weeks relieves eczema symptoms as well as such traditional treatments as lactic acid or urea. CBD oil is a great natural choice to soothe rashes and prevent flare-ups.

HOW TO USE

Apply CBD oil lotion generously to eczema rash 1–2 times daily. Avoid using CBD oil lotion with menthol or other drying agents.

77: SOOTHES BURNS

Most of us have experienced a nasty burn, whether it's from something as serious as a fire or something as small as touching a hot pan or spilling hot tea or coffee on our skin. Burns can be extremely painful for days and even weeks, and leave behind scars as they heal. One way to heal your burn and minimize any resulting scarring is by using a plant-based homemade remedy like CBD oil.

CBD oil can provide pain relief and wound healing as effective as or even more effective than commercial treatments that have synthetic ingredients you might not want your skin to absorb, especially if you've been burned in a sensitive region like the groin or face. CBD oil not only heals burns; it can also improve the quality of the unburned skinned around it. The natural ingredients in this CBD oil salve recipe accelerate burn healing by:

- Reducing inflammation.
- Fighting bacterial infections.
- Lessening pain.
- Increasing blood flow to the wound.
- Moisturizing dry skin.
- Shortening wound-healing time.

TO MAKE A CBD OIL BURN SALVE, COMBINE:

2 tablespoons extra virgin olive oil
¼ cup mānuka honey
15 drops lavender essential oil
5 drops peppermint essential oil
200 milligrams CBD oil

RECOMMENDATIONS FOR USE

Store in an airtight container at room temperature for up to four weeks. Apply generously to burn 1–2 times per day and cover with a bandage until fully healed.

78: FIGHTS GUM DISEASE

Gum disease (also known as periodontitis or periodontal disease) is a very common but painful condition that occurs when your gums recede and food gets trapped in pockets between your teeth and gums, causing bacteria to produce toxins that further inflame the gums. It's important to take care of your gums; if gum disease is left untreated, bone and gum tissue start to break down. Unhealthy gums can be a sign of poor health in general; the more inflamed your gums are, the more inflamed your body is overall. Patients with gum disease often have diabetes, heart disease, kidney disease, asthma, cancer, or one or more of over 120 other health conditions.

With over 47 percent of Americans experiencing such symptoms of periodontitis as bad breath and red, swollen, and bleeding gums, it's no wonder that people are searching for a natural way to stop gum damage. Peroxide and other ingredients in traditional toothpastes can irritate inflamed gums, which can turn toothbrushing into a painful nightmare.

CBD oil is a newer ingredient popping up in dental care products, and with good reason. CBD oil contains anti-inflammatory carrier oils, cannabinoids, and terpenes that all fight gum inflammation. Using CBD oil toothpaste can help freshen breath, fight bacteria and viruses, and save teeth from damage. Adding a ¼ of a dropper of CBD oil directly to your toothpaste and toothbrush is a quick and easy way to insert cannabinoids deep into the crevices of your gums. (Make sure to brush and rinse normally.) Another quick way to insert CBD oil into your gum care routine is by swishing CBD oil around in your mouth instead of just leaving it under your tongue before you swallow. Because CBD oil is absorbed both under the tongue (sublingual) as well as through the cheek (buccal), this method allows CBD oil to penetrate your gums while still being absorbed into your bloodstream.

79: PROMOTES HEALING OF COLD SORES

Cold sores are embarrassing and painful, but not uncommon. Over 50 percent of Americans have HSV-1 or HSV-2, the two types of herpes virus that can cause cold sores on the mouth. Some people with the virus show no symptoms, while others experience severe outbreaks of cold sores when triggered by feeling stress, drinking caffeine, or eating spicy foods. Topical and oral antiviral treatments are available via prescription and even OTC, but they can come with side effects such as headaches, nausea, and diarrhea that are as uncomfortable as the cold sores themselves.

Without intervention, cold sores can last four to seven days. Using such natural treatments as CBD oil can speed up the healing process and may even help cold sore outbreaks become less frequent. CBD oil contains phytocannabinoids and terpenes that kill viruses, reduce inflammation, and boost the immune system, making your body more effective at clearing the virus. CBD oil also works as an analgesic when applied topically, reducing throbbing pain and redness of the sores. Never apply a dropper full of CBD oil directly near your mouth or cold sore, however, as the contact could contaminate the rest of the bottle. Instead, make a separate jar of CBD oil cold sore cream, using the following recipe.

TO MAKE A COLD SORE CREAM, GATHER:

2 tablespoons beeswax

2 tablespoons organic coconut oil

½ tablespoon aloe vera gel

10 drops peppermint essential oil

6 drops tea tree essential oil

60 milligrams CBD oil

Heat beeswax and coconut oil in a small pot over low heat until liquid. Remove from heat and add aloe vera, essential oils, and CBD oil. Stir.

RECOMMENDATIONS FOR USE

Pour cream into a small tin and store at room temperature for up to twelve months. Apply to lips at first sign of cold sore symptoms 1–3 times daily for up to seven days. Do not share.

80: REDUCES BRUISING

Bruises can be a painful eyesore that take days if not weeks to heal. Some people bruise more than others, even if they don't bump into anything. Risk factors for bruising easily include drinking alcohol, having fair skin, being deficient in vitamin C or vitamin K, taking blood-thinning medications, or having a serious medical condition such as cancer, a bleeding disorder, or liver disease. While most people expect that time is the only remedy for bruises, there are natural treatments for bruising, including CBD oil.

Both eating CBD oil and applying it to your skin can heal bruising faster. CBD oil contains numerous anti-inflammatories, including quercetin, a flavonoid that prevents the release of histamines, which cause inflammation and swelling. CBD oil also contains antioxidants that can increase vitamin C levels in your body and strengthen blood vessels that are broken in the bruise. Whether you are ingesting CBD oil or using it as a topical, the choice of CBD oil product can influence the speed of your bruise healing. Choose a CBD oil that is green, as it has more plant matter in it than a CBD oil product that is clear. CBD oil that has a strong smell of grass may also include more vitamins

(such as vitamin K) that can heal bruises. You can also make your own inexpensive bruise-healing product at home with the following recipe.

TO MAKE A BRUISE-HEALING COMPRESS, GATHER:

1 teaspoon crushed fresh pineapple
15 milligrams CBD oil

Combine compress ingredients and apply to the bruise. Soak a hand towel in a bowl of hot water and then wring out the excess water. Lay the towel over compress ingredients and leave on for 20 minutes.

RECOMMENDATIONS FOR USE

Use as a hot compress daily for the first three days after bruising, and then use ice cold water instead of hot water for day four onward until the bruise has faded. Discard compress after each use.

81: ALLEVIATES DANDRUFF

Dandruff is a common but embarrassing condition that occurs when a naturally occurring fungus in your scalp overgrows, causing oil and skin cells on the scalp to flake off and dust white particles on your hair and clothes. In severe cases, dandruff can also cause itching and inflammation of the scalp. While the cause isn't exactly known, stress, use of some medications, and various medical conditions can trigger a dandruff flare-up. Regular use of shampoos containing harsh chemicals can often treat dandruff, but they can also strip hair dye or discolor naturally light hair. No matter what your hair color is, it can end up looking dry and brittle after using a synthetic dandruff shampoo.

CBD oil contains natural cannabinoids, terpenes, and fatty acids that can bring your scalp back into pH balance. CBD oil can moisturize dry skin, fight inflammation in the scalp, and stop the buildup of fungus that might cause dandruff. The end result is that your hair may look even better than it was before a dandruff episode. Use the following recipe for a natural CBD oil shampoo to beat dandruff and revitalize your hair in the process.

TO MAKE A CBD OIL DANDRUFF SHAMPOO, COMBINE:

2 tablespoons organic coconut oil
10 milligrams CBD oil
2 drops eucalyptus essential oil

RECOMMENDATIONS FOR USE

Wet hair and massage shampoo into it for 1 minute, avoiding the eyes. Leave on scalp for 2–3 minutes. Rinse thoroughly and let hair dry.

82: COMBATS SCARRING

Scars can be a constant reminder of past cuts, burns, acne, stretch marks, and surgeries. You will have the best results if you treat a wound right after it is made, but that requires repeated, consistent treatment to ensure the injury doesn't leave a mark. It's nearly impossible to fade a scar months or years after it's been formed unless it's lasered off, which can be expensive and require recovery time.

CBD oil contains hundreds of plant compounds that work together to boost the regeneration of healthy skin tissue—ingredients that put it ahead of commercial scar creams. Phytocannabinoids in CBD oil have the unique ability to boost the immune system and the secretion of chemicals that speed up healing. The ingredients in the following scar cream recipe all work to reduce the growth of scar tissue. They also boost circulation, decrease inflammation, relieve pain, moisturize skin, reduce hyperpigmentation, brighten dull skin, fight bacterial infection, and enhance shedding of dead skin cells.

TO MAKE A SCAR-REDUCING CREAM, COMBINE:

½ cup organic coconut oil
16 drops rosehip oil
6 drops tea tree essential oil
6 drops frankincense essential oil
8 drops lavender essential oil
50 milligrams CBD oil

RECOMMENDATIONS FOR USE

Store in an airtight jar at room temperature for up to eight weeks. Apply daily for two to three weeks for fresh wounds and up to sixteen weeks for older scars.

83: MOISTURIZES CRACKED LIPS

Dry, cracked lips can be painful as well as embarrassing. Whether it's from living in dry air, at high elevation, or through the blistering cold of winter, having cracked lips can expose you to bacteria, fungi, and viruses entering through the skin's tiny open wounds. Unfortunately, reaching for that menthol lip balm may not be your best bet, as most commercial lip balms are filled with chemicals that cause irritation and dry out your lips over the long run.

CBD oil is an amazingly effective ingredient for healing cracked lips. The phytocannabinoids in CBD oil reduce painful inflammation, and terpenes like limonene fight potential infections from bacteria and fungi. The medium-chain fatty acids in coconut oil moisturize lips and act as a barrier to protect them from wind and cold. By making the following CBD lip balm, you can heal your lips faster with natural ingredients and skip exposing yourself to toxins from commercial lip balm (which you would accidently swallow all day).

TO MAKE A CBD LIP BALM, GATHER:

¼ cup organic coconut oil

¼ cup shea butter

5 drops lavender essential oil

30 milligrams CBD oil

Melt coconut oil and shea butter together in microwave in 30-second increments until the mixture is a clear liquid. Add lavender and CBD oils, and mix. Pour into a tin and cool for 24 hours in the refrigerator before using.

RECOMMENDATIONS FOR USE

Store at room temperature for up to four weeks. Apply generously to lips as needed.

84: MAKES PAIN-RELIEVING BATH BOMB

Sometimes it hurts everywhere, and you simply can't coat your body head to toe in a pain-relieving lotion. That would be not only prohibitively expensive, it would also not be the quickest or most effective way to get relief for your aching muscles. By jumping in a hot bath and adding a CBD oil bath bomb, you can get essential minerals and oils into every inch of your body while achieving an ultimate state of bliss.

The following CBD bath bomb recipe contains potent ingredients that do the following:

- Calm tense muscles.
- Reduce inflammation.
- Relieve muscle pain.
- Relax the mind.
- Promote restorative sleep.

TO MAKE A CBD OIL BATH BOMB, GATHER:

¼ cup baking soda

2 tablespoons cornstarch

2 tablespoons citric acid

2 tablespoons Epsom salts

½ teaspoon water

1 teaspoon organic coconut oil

4 drops peppermint essential oil

4 drops lavender essential oil

25 milligrams CBD oil

Add baking soda, cornstarch, citric acid, and Epsom salts to a medium bowl and whisk together to remove clumps. Add remaining ingredients to another small bowl, soften in the microwave for 10–15 seconds, and mix. Slowly add the liquid mixture to the dry ingredient bowl while whisking. Slightly overfill each half of a metal bath bomb mold with mixture and press both halves together firmly for 5 seconds. Remove the top mold and let dry for 1 hour before flipping over and removing the bottom mold. Let bath bomb dry overnight.

RECOMMENDATIONS FOR USE

Wrap the bath bomb in foil or plastic wrap and keep away from moisture. Store at room temperature up to one year. Drop the bath bomb into a warm bath to enjoy.

85: SOOTHES ITCHY SKIN

When skin gets dry and inflamed, it gets itchy. And while some people are sensitive to triggers like scratchy fabrics, cold air, or chemicals in beauty products, others have medical conditions or take medications that make itchy skin a part of daily life. The drive to scratch itchy skin can make it worse, causing skin to dry out more and eventually peel. Commercial moisturizers and anti-itch products often smell unpleasant and are filled with synthetic chemicals that can actually make you itch more over the long term.

CBD oil is a natural treatment that can be applied directly to the skin as well as taken as a daily supplement to relieve and even prevent itchy skin—without costing a ton of money. CBD oil contains a bounty of phytocannabinoids, flavonoids, and terpenes that all work together to soothe and heal itchy skin when applied topically. Linalool, also found in lavender essential oil, is the most effective terpene for treating itchy skin. The main cannabinoid in CBD oil, CBD, increases activity of anandamide, an endocannabinoid that stimulates CB1 cannabinoid receptors in the skin to relieve itching as well as pain. When CBD oil is applied to the skin, it activates TRPV4 receptors in the skin to reduce inflammation. Whether you eat CBD oil or you apply a CBD oil cream to the skin, activating the endocannabinoid system has been found to calm mast cells (cells found in the tissue that are a key part of the immune system), reducing their release of histamines that cause inflammation and itching in the first place.

HOW TO USE

Lotions and creams with CBD oil and heavier ingredients like shea butter can be applied in the morning to provide a barrier against unavoidable irritants in your environment that can cause itchy skin. For best results, avoid using CBD oil products that contain additional synthetic or drying ingredients such as glycerin.

86: TACKLES BAD BREATH

Bad breath can be due to anything from eating a spicy or flavorful dinner, practicing bad dental hygiene, or even having a medical condition that may be undiagnosed. While brushing, flossing, and using mouthwash can cover up bad breath in some, for those who suffer from a chronic illness, having daily halitosis (chronic bad breath) is an embarrassing problem that doesn't seem to have an easy solution. Many of the mouthwashes, toothpastes, and gums on the market contain toxic chemicals that irritate and dry out the mouth, reducing saliva production and contributing to more bad breath in the long term.

For a natural solution, incorporate CBD oil into your daily dental cleaning routine. Containing phytocannabinoids that fight bacteria in the mouth that cause bad breath, CBD oil also moisturizes the mouth and reduces inflammation from prior exposure to harsh halitosis treatments. Combined with ginger (which contains a compound called gingerol that stimulates saliva to break down bad odors in your mouth), CBD oil can keep your breath fresh every day. The following recipe uses CBD oil and ginger for breath freshening and a tasty chew.

TO MAKE A BREATH FRESHENING CHEW, GATHER:

10 pieces dried ginger, chopped
100 milligrams CBD oil

Lay ginger pieces on parchment paper. Use a dropper to distribute CBD oil drops evenly on top of the ginger. Suck on or chew one CBD ginger chew for at least 1 minute to get full benefits. Store chews in an airtight container at room temperature for up to one year.

87: TARGETS ATHLETE'S FOOT

Athlete's foot can be an itchy nightmare, with a red, scaly rash starting in between your toes and spreading throughout your foot and even other parts of your body. Athlete's foot is contagious and can be caught by using the same towels or even walking on the same floor barefoot as someone who has it. OTC antifungal medications can kill the infection, but the harsh chemicals leave your feet susceptible to recurring infections.

Compared to commercial antifungal medications, CBD oil has triple the fungus-fighting power, with cannabinoids, terpenes, and coconut oil all being potent antifungals. Thankfully, CBD oil can also be used both internally and externally to treat athlete's foot much faster than other natural methods such as garlic or talcum powder. Use CBD oil daily as a tincture under the tongue to prevent recurrence of athlete's foot in people susceptible to chronic infections. The most powerful way to treat a current case of athlete's foot is to apply a treatment containing CBD oil directly to the foot. It's important not to just use a dropper of CBD oil on your feet, as the dropper might get contaminated with fungus, and the CBD oil won't penetrate as deeply into your foot as it would in a specially formulated cream. The following recipe has the ability to not only treat the underlying cause of athlete's foot, but also to naturally alleviate the resulting pain and inflammation.

TO MAKE CBD OIL ATHLETE'S FOOT CREAM, COMBINE:

1/8 cup aloe vera gel

1/8 cup organic coconut oil

8 drops tea tree essential oil

8 drops eucalyptus essential oil

60 milligrams CBD oil

RECOMMENDATIONS FOR USE

Store in an airtight container at room temperature for up to eight weeks. Massage into the foot (including between the toes) each night for up to four weeks until the infection heals.

88: MAKES A CALMING FACE MASK

Daily life is stressful, and unfortunately, that stress exacerbates skin issues. The signs of stress show up on our skin differently depending on our genes and body chemistry, and include blemishes, redness, puffiness, and uneven skin tone. Commercial skin treatments can often cause skin to become more irritated and out of balance, making natural treatments like CBD oil masks a better choice to calm stressed skin.

Skincare products containing CBD oil have phytocannabinoids that penetrate each layer of your skin to calm and balance. With additional benefits like fighting harmful bacteria, supporting healthy bacteria, and reducing excess sebum, cannabinoids and terpenes in CBD oil can help your skin go from a hot mess to glowing. Plus, taking the time to apply a face mask and press the pause button on life can give you a much-needed break in your stressful day, adding to the benefits of the mask ingredients. The following CBD face mask recipe contains powerful ingredients that:

- Calm redness.
- Reduce swelling.
- Fight free radicals.
- Hydrate the skin.
- Protect against sun damage.
- Reduce acne-causing bacteria.

TO MAKE A CALMING CBD FACE MASK, COMBINE:

1 teaspoon reishi mushroom powder
¼ teaspoon ground turmeric
1 tablespoon mānuka honey
3 drops lavender essential oil
25 milligrams CBD oil

RECOMMENDATIONS FOR USE

Use unflavored full-spectrum or broad-spectrum CBD oil if possible. Combine ingredients in a bowl and immediately apply mask to your face. After mask dries for 15 minutes, remove with a washcloth and warm water. Make fresh and use once a week to unwind and fight signs of stress.

89: COMBATS HAIR LOSS

There is perhaps nothing more terrifying than finding that your hair is falling out. The average person normally sheds fifty to one hundred strands of hair each day; losing more than that can be caused by severe stress, chronic illness, medications, and hormonal changes due to pregnancy or menopause. Alopecia, or balding, is the most severe form of hair loss that occurs in both women and men. Oral medications such as prednisone, and topical treatments such as minoxidil are commonly prescribed to stop hair thinning; but they often have dangerous side effects such as suppressing the immune system and impairing sexual function. Chemical-free remedies should be your first step, especially if you know your hair loss isn't due to a serious chronic illness.

CBD oil is a natural way to promote hair health and can be taken internally as well as added directly to the scalp. Taking CBD oil tincture daily can help relieve stress, which can prevent hair thinning. CBD oil applied to the scalp can add moisture, increase blood flow, and fight inflammation, securing the root of the hair follicle in place. The following recipe can be used at any time to strengthen your mane against potential hair loss.

TO MAKE A HEALING SCALP TREATMENT, COMBINE:

3 tablespoons softened organic coconut oil
4 drops rosemary essential oil
30 milligrams CBD oil

RECOMMENDATIONS FOR USE

Apply to scalp immediately and leave on for 10 minutes. Rinse out. Use weekly for healthy hair.

90: SOOTHES SORE NIPPLES

In theory, breastfeeding can be a beautiful bonding time between mother and child, but in reality, it may not go so easy when your newborn is first learning to breastfeed. Your baby biting too hard can cause dry, sore, cracked, and even bleeding nipples that can't heal because mealtimes are every couple of hours. While it might be tempting to reach for any old lotion or cream in your house, these remedies can expose your child to toxic chemicals like artificial dyes and fragrances that are in many common household beauty products.

One of the best ways to provide pain relief and prevent infections while keeping your child safe is to apply a natural cream or balm to the nipples between feedings. The plant-based nipple cream recipe that follows contains cannabinoids, terpenes, and fatty acids that:

- Soothe tender nipples.
- Moisturize and protect skin.
- Fight off bacterial infections.
- Don't expose your child to harmful ingredients.

Be sure to avoid products made with full-spectrum CBD oil and look for broad-spectrum CBD oil labeled "THC-Free" to prevent exposing your child to minute amounts of THC.

TO MAKE A NIPPLE BALM, COMBINE:

¼ cup extra virgin olive oil

½ cup organic coconut oil

2 tablespoons shea butter

6 drops lavender essential oil

25 milligrams CBD oil

RECOMMENDATIONS FOR USE

Store in an airtight jar at room temperature for up to two months. Begin applying daily the week before birth. Apply to nipples after breastfeeding. Wipe excess balm off nipples before breastfeeding again.

91: BALANCES OILY HAIR

Whether it's from sweat, multiple hair products, hormones, or bad genes, your hair can get oily and grimy fast. The excess oil on your scalp can clog pores, slow hair growth, and dry out the ends of your hair. Fortunately, taking 10–15 milligrams of CBD oil tincture every day can help balance your hormones and fight inflammation in hair follicles that may cause oily hair. CBD oil can also be applied topically to your scalp to prevent oily hair. The omega-3 and omega-6 fatty acids in CBD oil lock in moisture in your scalp, which prevents oil glands from overproducing oil. It may seem counterintuitive that adding CBD oil can help your hair be less oily; however, CBD's phytocannabinoids can promote cellular turnover in the scalp to prevent clogged pores. Additionally, antioxidants in CBD oil stop inflammation in the scalp, increase circulation, and improve the health of your hair.

When combined with essential oils, natural shampoo containing CBD can transform oily, stringy hair into shiny, voluminous locks. Use the following simple recipe to make your own inexpensive CBD shampoo.

TO MAKE A CBD OIL SHAMPOO, COMBINE:

1 cup distilled water
¼ cup liquid castile soap
1 tablespoon baking soda
6 drops peppermint essential oil
6 drops eucalyptus essential oil
50 milligrams CBD oil

RECOMMENDATIONS FOR USE

Store in an airtight jar at room temperature for up to eight weeks. Massage 2 teaspoons of shampoo into wet hair and rinse thoroughly.

92: MAKES AN ANTI-INFLAMMATORY TOOTHPASTE

Conventional toothpastes are filled with toxic chemicals such as artificial coloring, sodium fluoride, sodium lauryl sulfate, and glycerin that not only expose you to heavy metals but can also aggravate current inflammation in your gums and promote new inflammation. Applying liquids to your tongue and mouth is one of the fastest ways to absorb compounds in the body (it's why you place CBD oil under the tongue). Using a natural toothpaste is the only way to avoid absorbing those nasty chemicals straight into your bloodstream.

CBD oil's unique chemical profile makes it the perfect addition to natural toothpaste. Numerous cannabinoids and terpenes in CBD oil fight bacteria, virus, and fungus, keeping gum disease and even canker sores at bay. It's important to make your own CBD toothpaste at home, as products sold online are often made with the same toxic chemicals as traditional toothpaste. The following CBD toothpaste recipe contains potent ingredients with unique health benefits, including:

- Coconut oil: Fights bacteria and gum disease.
- Baking soda: Removes stains from teeth.
- CBD oil: Reduces pain and inflammation from mouth infections.

TO MAKE A CBD TOOTHPASTE, COMBINE:

4 tablespoons organic coconut oil

2 tablespoons baking soda

15 drops food-grade peppermint essential oil

60 milligrams CBD oil

RECOMMENDATIONS FOR USE

Store in an airtight jar at room temperature for up to two months. Use 2 times daily, once in the morning and once at night. Do not swallow.

93: AIDS TATTOO HEALING

More than 30 percent of Americans have at least one tattoo, and each one hopes to heal their new ink as quickly and painlessly as possible. Unfortunately, tattoos can take up to four weeks to heal, as the skin can scab and shed in response to the procedure. A well-healed tattoo will look fresh and clear for years to come, while a poorly healed tattoo can look cheap or improperly done.

Avoid applying moisturizers with synthetic chemicals to a tattoo, as the chemicals will be directly absorbed by the open wound into the bloodstream. CBD oil can be a safer, natural way to promote fast and proper tattoo healing, as it contains:

- Antioxidants that promote healthy blood flow.
- Anti-inflammatories that reduce redness and swelling.
- Antibacterial compounds that prevent infection.
- Fatty acids that moisturize the skin.
- Cannabinoids and terpenes that provide pain relief.

The essential oils and coconut oil in the following tattoo balm support the delivery of healing CBD oil compounds to the deep layers of the skin.

TO MAKE A TATTOO BALM, COMBINE:

2 tablespoons organic coconut oil

5 drops lavender essential oil

5 drops tea tree essential oil

20 milligrams CBD oil

RECOMMENDATIONS FOR USE

Store in an airtight container in the refrigerator for up to one month. Apply balm before receiving your tattoo and daily afterward for one week. Covering with a bandage or gauze is optional.

94: FIGHTS NAIL INFECTIONS

Billions of dollars are spent each year on keeping nails beautifully manicured, but salons can be a source of germs that cause both nail infections and small skin tears that let those germs enter the body. Because nail infections can be extremely painful and embarrassing for many, a treatment that is inexpensive but acts fast is a must. Unfortunately, most OTC treatments for nail infections are made with synthetic chemicals that cause burning and irritation, further harming nail health. Luckily, CBD oil is a great alternative to help prevent and treat nail infections.

CBD oil is effective at fighting both the bacteria and fungus that can cause nail infections. Many of the phytochemicals in CBD oil are both antifungal and antibacterial, including the terpenes beta-caryophyllene and limonene, and cannabinoids CBD, CBG, and CBC. The most common carrier oil for CBD oil is MCT oil, which is made from coconut oil and has antifungal properties itself. CBD oil also contains anti-inflammatory compounds that can reduce pain and promote the healing of nail infections.

CBD oil can be taken daily as a tincture to reduce growth of bacteria and fungus in the body, which can prevent nail infections. It can also be used topically to help prevent and treat nail infections. A dose of 10 milligrams is recommended.

TO MAKE AN ANTIFUNGAL NAIL TREATMENT, COMBINE:

1 tablespoon organic coconut oil

2 drops tea tree essential oil

2 drops eucalyptus essential oil

10 milligrams CBD oil

RECOMMENDATIONS FOR USE

Store in an airtight container at room temperature for up to two weeks. Apply to your nails the day before and after visiting a nail salon or daily when experiencing symptoms of a nail infection.

95: HYDRATES CRACKED HEELS

Winter can leave your feet dry and your heels cracked. And if you have a medical condition like diabetes or psoriasis that dries out your skin or slows wound healing, you might deal with cracked heels year-round. While cracked heels are embarrassing to many, they can also be painful and even dangerous for your health, as bacteria, fungus, and even viruses can enter the open wounds. Heels that are cracked are slow to heal and require daily TLC with natural remedies to revitalize your feet.

CBD oil has phytocannabinoids and terpenes that fight microbes, moisturize skin, and boost circulation, helping cracked heels mend faster. Use the following CBD oil heel repair mask anytime as a healing moisturizer for your feet.

TO MAKE A CBD HEEL REPAIR MASK, COMBINE:

1 cup organic coconut oil

2 teaspoons cocoa butter

1 teaspoon lemon juice

2 tablespoons pure honey

3 drops lavender essential oil

150 milligrams CBD oil

RECOMMENDATIONS FOR USE

Soak feet in warm water for 20 minutes and dry with a towel before applying the mask to feet. Massage mask into each foot, applying a thicker layer to the heels. For best results, apply before bedtime, cover with cotton socks, and leave on while sleeping. Remove socks and rinse with warm water without soap the next day. Use 3–5 times per week until heels have healed. Store in an airtight jar at room temperature for up to four weeks.

96: COMBATS PSORIASIS

Psoriasis is a common but embarrassing skin condition that is characterized by red, itchy patches and scales that can be painful. It is caused by skin cells growing and shedding too quickly, resulting in a buildup of dry skin cells. While scientists don't know exactly what causes psoriasis, we do know that your immune system, genetics, and lifestyle can affect whether you develop the condition and how severe flare-ups can be.

If you are one of the eight million Americans who experience psoriasis, you can help treat and even prevent flare-ups with CBD oil. Cannabinoids in CBD oil, including CBD, CBG, and CBN, were found to slow down the growth of skin cells in the outer layer of the skin as well as lessen their production of keratins, proteins that normally form the waterproof protective barrier of skin. CBD oil is also anti-inflammatory and relieves itching and pain, meaning it works fast to get you back to feeling and looking like your best.

TO MAKE A PSORIASIS SALVE, GATHER:

¼ cup aloe vera gel
¼ cup softened organic coconut oil
500 milligrams CBD oil
15 drops tea tree essential oil
10 drops geranium essential oil

Whisk together aloe vera and coconut oil in a medium bowl. Add in remaining oils and stir.

RECOMMENDATIONS FOR USE

Store in an airtight jar in the refrigerator for up to one month. Apply generously to skin as needed for psoriasis relief.

97: MAKES SOOTHING BODY SCRUB

When you are stressed out or sleep deprived, your outer state starts to reflect your inner tension; your skin gets dry, irritated, and slow to shed. And when you don't look your best, it makes it even harder to feel your best. Layering moisturizers and body balms can help with the dryness, but these are just temporary solutions. Instead, kickstart your healing journey by scrubbing away tiredness and stress and indulging in some self-care by exfoliating your skin.

CBD oil is an essential ingredient in a body scrub because of the hundreds of plant compounds that work together to improve the health of your mind, body, and soul. The following CBD body scrub helps your skin go from grimy to glowing in no time with ingredients that:

- Stimulate circulation and flush away toxins.
- Moisturize skin.
- Relieve pain and inflammation.
- Relax tense muscles.
- Calm your mind.

TO MAKE A SOOTHING CBD SCRUB, COMBINE:

½ cup organic coconut oil
½ cup granulated sugar
4 drops peppermint essential oil
12 drops lavender essential oil
30 milligrams CBD oil

RECOMMENDATIONS FOR USE

Massage scrub in circular patterns over skin to shed dead skin cells and stimulate circulation. Use 1–2 times per week. Store in an airtight jar at room temperature for up to four weeks.

98: PROMOTES HAIR GROWTH

Everyone wants shiny, strong hair with lots of volume, but everything from genetics to a poor diet can keep us far away from that goal. Thankfully, there are natural ways to speed up hair growth, including using CBD oil. When taken daily as a tincture, CBD oil adds antioxidants and anti-inflammatories to your system that increase blood flow and promote keratin to build new hair. CBD oil also contains omega-3 fatty acids that relieve inflammation and speed hair growth. When CBD oil is applied directly to the hair, the fatty acids in the oil moisturize and repair damage to the hair shaft, keeping growing hair strong.

Instead of buying expensive hair care brands in the store, save money and ensure all-natural ingredients (and no chemicals) by making your own CBD oil shampoos and conditioners at home. Because THC directly activates CB1 receptors in the scalp and slows hair growth, choose a broad-spectrum CBD oil without THC for DIY shampoos and conditioners.

TO MAKE A CBD CONDITIONER, COMBINE:

4 tablespoons organic coconut oil
2 tablespoons aloe vera gel
8 drops rosemary essential oil
30 milligrams CBD oil

RECOMMENDATIONS FOR USE

Apply to the scalp and massage into hair for 5 minutes. Let it sit for 10 minutes and then rinse. Store in an airtight container at room temperature for up to eight weeks and use once a week.

99: FIGHTS TOOTH DECAY

That piece of food stuck in between your teeth breaks down into sugar, feeding bacteria in your mouth and combining with saliva to form plaque. Plaque turns into tartar, a layer of bacteria that weakens tooth enamel by removing minerals from it. Cavities form when softened enamel creates openings that bacteria dive into and further break down the inside layer of the tooth (called the dentin), causing serious tooth pain. Thankfully, you can fight tooth decay before it turns into a full-blown cavity with CBD oil.

CBD oil contains phytocannabinoids that kill bacteria in your mouth, preventing plaque from forming. They also fight inflammation and increase blood flow, slowing down tooth decay that is already in progress. Finally, CBD oil is alkaline, so it can offset the effect of acidic foods like coffee and juice that damage your tooth enamel. CBD oil is safe to use in your mouth and beneficial to swallow. You can use CBD oil every day to clean and protect your teeth, either by making a natural toothpaste with CBD oil, or adding several drops of CBD oil to your toothbrush along with your regular toothpaste, and brushing as normal to get the benefits of using CBD oil for oral hygiene.

100: SOOTHES SUNBURNS

Sunburns are an inevitable part of life for many. You're more vulnerable to sunburn if you live in a city located at a higher altitude, work outdoors for a living, or spend a lot of time on the beach. No matter how it happens, sunburn can damage DNA in your skin, causing skin redness, pain, and peeling. This DNA damage can lead to premature skin aging; a severe sunburn or multiple moderate sunburns can also lead to skin cancer.

It's important to protect your skin by healing sunburns as swiftly and properly as possible, and by preventing future sunburns. CBD oil is a natural solution for sunburn relief. CBD has more powerful antioxidant activity than vitamin C or vitamin E, and all three are found in CBD oil and act to fight free-radical damage in your skin. CBD oil also contains terpenes such as linalool that reduce redness and swelling by acting as anti-inflammatory compounds. Phytocannabinoids in CBD oil can relieve pain naturally. Finally, carrier oils such as coconut oil found in CBD oil can moisturize sunburned skin and prevent itching and peeling of the skin. Add CBD oil to your favorite natural sunburn treatment to reduce the consequences of staying in the sun too long while improving the look and feel of your skin.

TO MAKE AN AFTER-SUN LOTION, GATHER:

$1/8$ cup aloe vera gel
$1/8$ cup softened organic coconut oil
250 milligrams CBD oil
8 drops lavender essential oil

Whisk together aloe vera and coconut oil in a medium bowl. Add in remaining oils and stir.

RECOMMENDATIONS FOR USE

Store in an airtight jar in the refrigerator for up to one month. Apply to skin immediately after sun exposure and as often as necessary to provide sunburn relief.

APPENDIX: SOURCING CBD OIL

You can find CBD oil online, in CBD stores, and even at gas stations, but how do you know that the CBD oil you are buying is safe or effective? The lack of government regulations on CBD oil means it is up to the consumer to do their research before buying a product. There are several questions you need to have answered before you purchase your CBD oil:

- Is the CBD oil full-spectrum, broad-spectrum, or isolate?
- What is the dose of CBD in the bottle (milligrams/milliliters)?
- Is the CBD oil third-party lab tested for pesticides or heavy metals?
- Where is the CBD oil produced?
- Are the other ingredients safe and effective?
- Is the brand of CBD oil trustworthy?

All of these questions can be easily answered on the product's website. CBD oil should not be an impulse buy. You will be able to determine if a CBD oil brand is reputable if it is made with hemp grown in the United States, and if it has a recent third-party lab test available to show that it is safe to consume and that it contains the amount of CBD oil listed on the bottle. Deciding whether a CBD oil brand is trustworthy can feel tricky at first, but transparency of information and lack of illegal medical claims on the website and package are good indicators of a reputable brand. Claims that CBD oil cures cancer or will help you lose 10 pounds in two weeks are not only false—they're illegal. A reputable company will also answer any questions you have about the brand promptly via email and phone, and will have testimonials or reviews by real customers on their website.

Quality Brands

The following are examples of brands that meet the standards for safe and effective CBD products. While full-spectrum CBD oil products may be marginally more effective for symptom relief than broad-spectrum CBD oil products, you may want to go with THC-free broad-spectrum CBD oil products if there is a possibility of being drug-tested.

Healist Naturals

Healist Naturals provides broad-spectrum CBD oil products formulated with clinically effective levels of organic botanical ingredients. Their products are THC-free.

https://healistnaturals.com

Veriheal

Veriheal connects patients with medical professionals that provide personalized telehealth consults in all fifty US states.

www.veriheal.com

Charlotte's Web

Created by the Stanley Brothers, Charlotte's Web is one of the original full-spectrum CBD oil brands, and has a 20:1 ratio of CBD to THC.

www.charlottesweb.com

Quality Care

It's important to note who is qualified to provide you with advice about using CBD oil for health and wellness purposes. Most CBD oil brand representatives and retail store employees lack medical training. For an objective and qualified opinion, it's best to talk to a doctor, nurse, or health coach who is specifically trained in using CBD oil. The following is an example of a trusted online service for CBD oil consultations.

INDEX

100 Delicious Recipes
for Total Mind and Body Wellness!

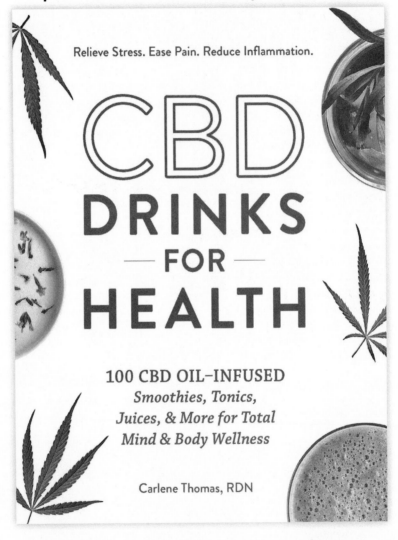

Relieve Stress. Ease Pain. Reduce Inflammation.

CBD
DRINKS
— FOR —
HEALTH

100 CBD OIL–INFUSED
*Smoothies, Tonics,
Juices, & More for Total
Mind & Body Wellness*

Carlene Thomas, RDN

Pick Up or Download Your Copy Today!

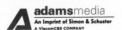

adamsmedia
An Imprint of Simon & Schuster
A ViacomCBS COMPANY